# Modern Psychiatry: Challenges in Educating Health Professionals to Meet New Needs





*A Conference Sponsored by the Josiah Macy, Jr. Foundation*

*Chaired by Beatrix Hamburg, M.D.*

*Toronto Canada*
*October 26-28, 2001*

*Edited by Mary Hager*

*Published by the*
*Josiah Macy, Jr. Foundation*
*44 East 64th Street*
*New York, NY 10021*

*2002*

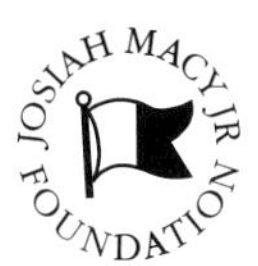

# Table of Contents

# Preface

## Dedication of Macy Conference

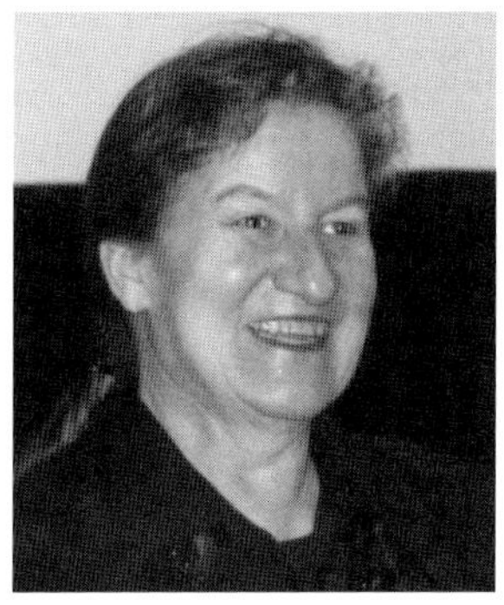

**June E. Osborn, M.D., President,**
**The Josiah Macy Jr. Foundation**
**October 26, 2001**

I am pleased to welcome you to this Macy Conference on "Modern Psychiatry: Challenges in Educating Health Professionals to Meet New Needs." Our goal is an ambitious one — to look for and recommend opportunities to ensure that the education of professionals in mental health fields is appropriate and adequate to the future needs of the United States.

I am deeply grateful to Dr. Betty Hamburg for having accepted my invitation to serve as the Chairwoman of this endeavor. She has provided committed and creative leadership in composing a remarkable planning committee and then in bringing such an impressive group of conferees together; and I am confident that she will lead us toward a set of recommendations and conclusions that can be helpful to future planning of educational strategies.

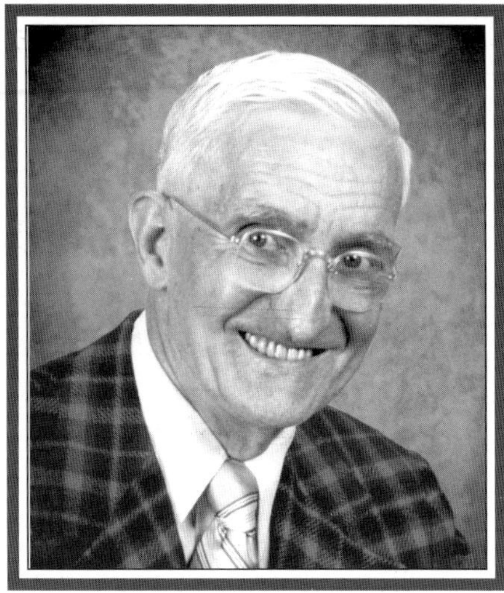

*Dr. Leslie A. Osborn*

Before I get to that, though, I want to take a few minutes of personal privilege. First, I would like to introduce to you my sister, Dr. Anne Osborn Krueger, currently on leave from her position as Professor of Economics at Stanford University. I am delighted that she is here to join me in dedicating this conference to our late father, Dr. Leslie A. Osborn, whose passion for and dedication to psychiatry and medicine was extraordinary. On September 1 of this year, Anne took leave from Stanford to become First Deputy Director of the International Monetary Fund. Given the rigors of that position I am particularly grateful that she persevered in her intent to take precious time from her duties in Washington, and for that matter around the world, to be with us today.

Our father was one of the most passionately committed clinicians I have known, and one of the most ardent teachers of psychiatry as well. Briefly, he earned his medical degree from the University of Melbourne, Australia, did an internship and then, in 1931, emigrated to North America with our mother Dora Emma Wright, his new bride. They landed in New York State in the depths of the depression. After a rocky start, for a number of years he was a general practitioner for the Endicott-Johnson Shoe Company in upstate New York, in which context he became convinced that interpersonal relationships and problems played pivotal, indeed determinative, roles in human health.

Ultimately he decided to do psychiatric training, ending up at the beginning of World War II on the University of Buffalo Medical School faculty; and indeed he became chairman of its Department of Psychiatry in the late 1940s. From there he went on to Wisconsin where he became both Director of the Division of Mental Hygiene for the State and Professor of Psychiatry in the Medical School.... to go much further would overstretch your indulgence. Suffice to say that he was a lover of humanity, an enthusiast about English literature, an iconoclast, a non-Freudian in an era where that was almost lethal academically, and a true genius when it came to one-on-one therapy of troubled people. I wish he were here to vent his feelings about manuals — he might well applaud the broadening of access that they surely represent — but his inventive soul would recoil at the notion that interpersonal dynamics could be so systematized. He was, above all, a role model in psychotherapeutics. A remarkable number of his former residents at the University of Buffalo came together fifty years after their training to celebrate his impact on their clinical lives.

One other feature of his wonderful persona should be mentioned: he was as tolerant a person as I have ever known. Such tolerance took many forms. For instance, when AIDS came along and had special, initial impact on gay communities throughout the country, many people were truly ignorant about their plight. I found, however, that I didn't need to give him an explication – he already understood.

The value of each human life was central to his being and played an important role in my sister's and my lives growing up. Perhaps nowhere did that count more than in his attitude to women. If you know about Australia, England and Empire, you can guess that he grew up in a framework of male chauvinism that occasionally bent but did not break. But he defied it. Our mother was an exceedingly bright, talented woman whom he supported fully in her endeavors. From a Tasmanian farm background til the age of 10, she nonetheless excelled in studies and had already earned a master's degree in early childhood education from the University of Hobart when he met her in 1927.

After they married and moved to the United States, where she pursued a successful junior faculty career in that field, someone persuaded her in the 1940s that women didn't get PhDs, and nepotism laws blocked her progress at the University of Wisconsin. So she reenrolled when I was in high school and ended up with two masters' degrees, the second in psychiatric social work. She distinguished herself memorably in both fields before her premature death in 1960. And my sister and I never wondered, for a minute, whether we would get a graduate education, only in what field. Anne went into economics (which has sometimes prompted her to introduce herself, in my company, as the "black sheep" of the family) while I opted for medicine.

So his legacy was very potent: in essence he was the greatest supporter, the most ardent clinician, the most passionate advocate of human worth I have ever known. To him, everyone was special. The great pediatrician, Dr. Edwards Park of Johns Hopkins Medical School, once described to me a former student of his, a wonderful woman physician, as someone "...into whose presence you enter feeling like the most ordinary of ducklings, but leave feeling like the most magnificent of swans." Dad had that quality too.

When our father died in the summer of 1996, Anne and I agreed that his commitment to psychiatry and to the people in need of its care should be honored in some way. I suppose the idea was lurking in the back of my head when I became President of the Macy Foundation a few months later, but in fact the idea of a Macy Conference on the future of psychiatry surfaced afterwards and for other reasons. Thanks to Dr. David Lewis, I became quite involved with efforts to deal with substance abuse and addiction. In that context I became aware that arcane public policy debates about "parity" were on-going. To encapsulate the central theme of those arguments: the issue was whether mental illness (and substance abuse, in tandem) really were worthy of necessary treatment and care and therefore qualified for health insurance coverage, or whether they were in some way "boutique" problems, to be dealt with or "topped off" if one could afford it. Having grown up knowing that mental illness was, for sure, illness, I was startled at the inferred disparity. To me, psychiatric care was integral to medicine, and the mind/body dichotomy was an astonishing intellectual construct that served to excuse physicians from the duty to care for illness, whatever the sort.

Then I came upon a fascinating book by T. H. Luhrmann, called Of Two Minds: the Growing Disorder in American Psychiatry. In it she gave an account of having trailed along, as an anthropologist, for a number of years, following psychiatric residents during their training. It was her observation that they were, in essence, being trained to two disparate roles — as psychopharmacologists and as psycho-therapists — with little adhesion between those different and yet potentially synergistic approaches. It seemed to me that a crisis might be at hand — in the classic Chinese calligraphic sense of combined danger + opportunity, and so the idea for the Macy Conference was born.

The central goal of the Macy Foundation is to find ways to improve health professional education, and I hope during these two-and-a-half days, as we explore the current situation of mental health, mental illness and the professions that seek to enhance the former and prevent or treat the latter, that we will bring into focus repeatedly the educational issues that might improve circumstances. We want, at the end of our deliberations, to achieve a consensus on a set of recommendations that will meet those objectives, and indeed the last half day will be devoted to arriving at such agreement, which will then be represented both in an executive summary and, later, in a monograph. I am particularly grateful to Ms. Mary Hager for her ongoing and anticipated role in those endeavors – she has been present in our planning meetings, and she is a diligent listener and a wonderful rapporteur whose notes have clarified many a cloudy discussion in the past and will surely do so here. I also want to introduce to you – face to face — the wonderful Macy Foundation staff who have so ably brought us to this juncture: Martha Wolfgang, our vice-president; and Tashi Dakar Ridley and Tanya Tyler, our respective assistants.

In conclusion, then, let me dedicate our deliberations and forthcoming recommendations to the memory of Dr. Leslie A. Osborn, whose passionate commitment to psychiatry and medicine can serve as inspiration in our task.

I now turn the podium over to Betty Hamburg, our leader, who will begin the proceedings.

June E. Osborn MD

# Foreword

## Modern Psychiatry: Challenges in Educating Health Professionals to Meet New Needs

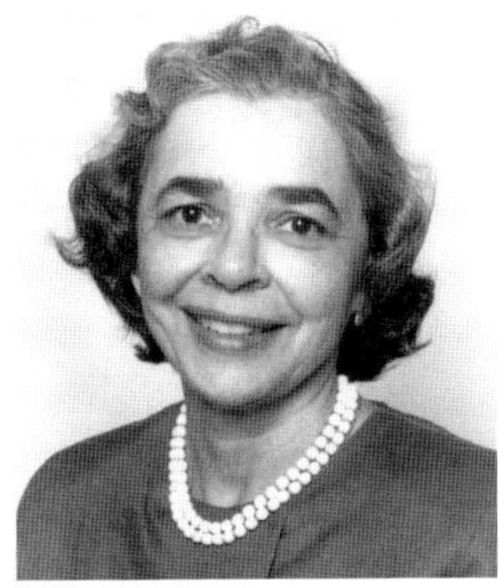

**Beatrix Hamburg, M.D.**

> "We must capitalize on this, the most exciting time in the history of biology..... We owe it to our patients"
> — *Steven Hyman, (Josiah Macy,Jr. Conference, October 2001)*

This clarion call signals the fact that as we enter the 21st century, it is timely and important to foster the development of a new era in the delivery of high quality mental health services to the large and growing population of persons with mental disorders in America. Among the many issues confronting modern psychiatry, the need for serious attention to the recruitment, education and training of mental health professionals for new roles and with new skills is essential. In planning the conference, this task was seen to fit well with the long-standing mission of the Josiah Macy, Jr. Foundation to improve the training of health professionals. It is also highly compatible with stirrings within a number of the relevant professions to assess and revise their training goals and curricula for current and future practitioners. This conference explores the challenges and opportunities in setting an agenda to address the gap between the advances in the science base and current clinical education and practices.

The remarkable scientific achievements of the latter part of the 20th century that pertain to mental health include advances in molecular and cognitive neuroscience, genetics and other biomedical sciences, behavioral and social sciences. Taken together, they constitute the exciting new neurobiology of brain and behavior. Much of the excitement derives from the demonstration of significant linkages and interactions across all of these domains. Mental health science is now interdisciplinary at all levels. Over the past decade this modern neurobiology has led to a transformation in fundamental concepts about psychiatric disorders. It is recognized that there is no single, simple explanation for a serious mental disorder, whether it be a gene or a specific biochemical process. In turn, over the past decade there has been greater appreciation of the importance of rigorous clinical research as a key contributor to the advancement of mental health science. In this, as in other areas of neuroscience, the technological advances in neuroimaging have played a critical role. It is now possible to image the living, functioning brain and trace the brain sites and neural circuits of a clinical response. Collaborations between basic scientists and rigorous clinicians are now recognized as vital to furthering insights about the mechanisms linking behavior and brain function.

There can be no doubt that the brain is a dynamic, malleable organ that alters in response to environmental stimuli, social interactions and social context. Increasingly there is knowledge about the nature of some systematic changes in brain structure and function, for example, responses during sensitive developmental periods, effects of emotion on learning and the cumulative impacts of aggregated stress. Appreciation of the multifactorial nature of brain-behavior interactions also heightens the need to understand more about the key elements in the social environment that either trigger adverse brain responses or buffer the individual.

While there is no expectation that all relevant mental health professionals will be expected to master the vast and complex literature of modern neurobiology, it is important that the basic findings, the conceptual framework, and relevance for clinical expertise be understood and that this science base be translated into their education and clinical training.

Surprisingly, important advances over the past 15 years in evidence-based psychotherapy (EBT) have received relatively scant attention. At this time, evidence-based treatments exist for the full spectrum of psychiatric disorders. Most psychotherapy is delivered by psychiatrists, psychologists and social workers. EBT is primarily intended for these practitioners The criteria for designation of psychotherapy as EBT are clear and rigorous. They include: prior clinical research validation of efficacy of the treatment by controlled clinical trial; careful diagnosis; specification of core elements of the therapy and treatment procedures in a manual and specification of therapist training requirements and procedures in a manual. Typically, these treatments are time limited. They have proven to be reliable and effective.

In other research, controlled clinical trials comparing the relative efficacy of psychotherapy and pharmacotherapy for the treatment of depression have shown that EBT is equal in efficacy with antidepressant drugs. Further, in many instances, combined EBT and drug therapy has been found to be more effective than either one alone. Recently, there has been great interest in brain imaging studies that analyzed brain function in patients with obsessive-compulsive disorder treated with EBT or SSRI drugs (selective serotonin reuptake inhibitors). Patients who responded positively to treatment, whether EBT or drugs, showed virtually the same brain changes when examined with PET brain scans. Both, along with their clinical improvement, showed decrease of hyperactivity in the caudate nucleus. When similar neuroimaging studies of brain responses were performed with depressed patients treated with either EBT or SSRI medication, PET scans showed that patients who improved showed functional brain changes in other specific areas of the brain that were virtually the same regardless of whether the improvement was brought about by EBT psychotherapy or SSRI medication. Although this comparability of effect on brain function was confirmed for depression, further studies are needed to establish the generalizability of the extent of the phenomenon across the range of psychiatric diagnoses. This promising line of research depends on continuing collaboration between neuroscientists and clinical investigators trained in pharmacotherapy and evidence-based psychotherapy.

In 1999 a ground-breaking *Report of the Surgeon-General on Mental Health* was issued by Surgeon-General David Satcher. In his own words, this science-based comprehensive document represents, "A Vision for the Future: Actions for Mental Health in the New Millennium". The report documents the efficacy of a broad range of available, evidence based mental health treatments. It highlights the heavy personal and societal burden of mental illness and the urgency of treating and preventing mental disorders and calls attention to those groups for whom there are notable and conitinuing disparities in mental health care. There was heavy emphasis on mental health services and mental health providers.

This Josiah Macy, Jr. conference reflects the spirit and the substance of Dr. Satcher's worthy goals and represents our efforts to begin the process of setting an agenda for the tasks of educating and training a new generation of mental health professionals. Our conference goals were to review the salient research advances, to specify the evidence base for new or modified service delivery, to delineate the spectrum of contemporary service needs, to make concrete recommendations to redesign the education and training of an appropriate mental health professional workforce.

An interdisciplinary group of outstanding leaders in their respective fields was convened for a three day invitational conference. The group of 34 invitees included: adult, child, and geriatric psychiatry; internal medicine; pediatrics; nursing; social work; psychology; public health; neuroscience; mental health, health administration; school psychology; health economics; social psychology; clinical psychology; epidemiology; history of medicine; public school administration. Six group members prepared commissioned papers. These were distributed to the entire group to be read prior to the conference. The authors gave brief highlights of their papers at the meeting. The full texts of these papers are printed in this monograph. Eight other participants were invited to give brief presentations in areas of their expertise. Edited versions of these remarks are also included in the monograph. The conference was divided into five sessions. The comments of the distinguished invited participants were viewed as a valuable contribution and ample time for discussion was allocated at each session. Discussion comments for each session are part of the monograph. One participant agreed to the daunting task of summarizing highlights of the entire wide ranging meeting. The text of his superb statement is printed in full. Following those remarks, the conference concluded with group discussion. Out of all this rich material, conclusions and recommendations were generated.

It has been a pleasure to work with Dr. June Osborn. I want to give special thanks to her for the opportunity to chair this important conference, one that also has personal significance for her. It is an honor to participate in paying tribute to her distinguished father. I also want to express my appreciation to the Planning Committee for their dedicated efforts. The staff of the Josiah Macy, Jr. Foundation has lightened all our tasks through their hard work and unfailing good cheer. I am deeply grateful to: Tashi Dakar Ridley, Tanya Tyler, Martha Wolfgang and to Mary Hager for her editing expertise. I also want to thank my secretary Mary Ferguson for her valuable assistance.

The conference was planned in the early part of the year 2001. However, it was held in October, 2001 in the immediate aftermath of the terrorist attacks of September 11. When we met it was already apparent that, in addition to the destruction and loss of life, the toll of mental health casualty was of massive proportions. There was an unprecedented demand for mental health services. There was widespread depression, post traumatic stress, and severe anxiety among those who had never experienced acute mental distress previously. For others, there were flare-ups and recurrences of prior symptoms that had been in remission. Over the ensuing months there has been a realization that the mental distress and disorders were not transient as had been expected by some. There are long-term mental health needs as a result of the 9/11 disaster. The anthrax scares and the continuing rainbow-colored terrorist alerts contribute to a national "Age of Anxiety" of unknown duration. The need to recruit and train mental health professionals has taken on a new urgency.

Beatrix A. Hamburg, M.D.

# Chairman's Summary of the Conference

Macy Foundation President June E. Osborn, M.D., dedicated the conference to the memory of her father, the late Leslie A. Osborn, M.D., a professor of psychiatry and clinician who had, she recalled, "passion for and dedication to psychiatry and medicine."

## The Context

Most Americans are aware of the spectacular health gains achieved during the 20th century in combating medical illness and extending the life span by 30 years, but there is far less appreciation for the remarkable scientific progress that dramatically and fundamentally changed the understanding of mental illness and its treatment over that same period.

One hundred years ago, because of ignorance, those with mental illness were feared and demonized. Patients were stigmatized, considered untreatable, and isolated in remote asylums. Psychoanalysis was launched in Europe early in the century and fairly soon began to flourish in America, providing the basis for a humane and psychodynamic approach to understanding patient concerns and behaviors. This understanding was based on life history and the observed attitudes and discussions from therapeutic sessions.

At mid-century, the approach to treatment added a new dimension as new medications were discovered that were highly effective in treating some of the most seriously disturbed patients. With these medications, many previously untreatable patients could be discharged and returned to the community though appropriate care and supervision of many of these patients was a problem, and continues to be today. Overall, these drugs constituted a major clinical breakthrough and the new field of psychopharmacology grew to include seminal studies of how these psychoactive drugs influence the brain. As a result of ongoing research, new and more effective drugs with fewer adverse side effects continue to be produced. For many years the treatment pathways of psychodynamic therapy and psychopharmacology diverged, but eventually the value of their combined use became well established.

The burgeoning of neuroscience, cognitive science, behavioral and social sciences, genetics, molecular biology and neuroimaging during the last quarter of the 20th century produced what many consider the most exciting and important area of human biology. A series of informative findings from research and interdisciplinary studies across these fields transformed the understanding of mental illness, disclosed linkages with medical illness, and provided detailed knowledge of brain functions, and mechanisms and structures involved in mental illness. New clues about the genetic and environmental factors that influence brain structure and function were uncovered, producing surprising new insights about brain responsiveness and plasticity. The integrated approach to neuroscience research facilitated rigorous systematic approaches to developing new psychodynamic, psychopharmacologic and psychosocial treatments for mental illness. The 1999 Report of the Surgeon-General on Mental Health states: "The efficacy of mental health treatments is well-documented and a range of treatments exists for most mental disorders." That is very good news.

Nonetheless, in the words of Leon H. Eisenberg, M.D., "Psychiatry is in the paradoxical position of having much more effective treatments to offer and of being much less able to provide them." This failure to provide effective treatment is of deep concern because in the United States mental illness is the second leading cause of disability and premature death, second only to all cardiovascular diseases. Mental disorders collectively account for more than 15 percent of the burden of illness from all causes.

Availability of treatment for mental disorder has acquired new urgency since the tragic events of September 11 and the anthrax bioterrorist attacks. The powerful impacts of these events in causing severe and widespread continuing mental distress and disorders have been a revelation. Existing facilities have proven inadequate to meet either the needs of the new cases or the heightened needs of those whose preexisting mental disorders were reactivated by the disaster.

## The Conference

What are some of the barriers to the delivery of proven effective treatments?

The primary focus of the Macy conference was on the notable lag in the translation of the scientific knowledge and advances in the diagnosis and treatment of mental disorders into the education and training of the spectrum of relevant health professionals. In addition, the significant shortages in mental health personnel were a key concern. The most critical needs are for the treatment of children and adolescents and to recruit minority persons to the mental health professions. Closely related are issues of education and training for the paraprofessionals who work in the various components of the poorly coordinated mental health system.

Significant other contributing factors were considered, but not discussed in detail. In addition to inequities and financial barriers within the medical system (Medicaid, Medicare and HMOs), as noted in the Report of the Surgeon-General, these included the complex, poorly integrated "system" of public and private social service agencies, the criminal justice system, schools and faith-based organizations and the problems of access, financing and patient frustration which are significant disincentives to seeking or remaining in care.

Although it has steadily decreased over recent years, stigma remains a problem for the mentally ill and can be a deterrent to obtaining treatment. Public ignorance of signs and symptoms of mental disorder along with lack of awareness of the fact that effective treatments do exist, can also contribute to the failure to seek available and effective care.

Commissioned papers, prepared remarks and general discussion were integral parts of the conference. The opening session provided an overview of the full range of issues confronting the field, including a review of the dominant themes in psychiatry during the 20th century, the growing role of epidemiology in rigorously defining the nature and scope of the psychiatric population, and an outline of the organization and financing of the health care system as well as issues of the size and composition of the mental health professional workforce. Subsequent sessions targeted areas of special interest for more in depth exploration: children and adolescents, the elderly, substance abuse as a dual diagnosis, minority groups and poverty in relation to mental health. After two and a half days, participants, who had been selected to provide expertise across a variety of perspectives, agreed upon the recommendations found at the end of this summary. As was clear from the recommendations, meeting the challenge of educating mental health professionals to meet future needs will require a coordinated effort by all those involved in and concerned about mental health, including consumers and advocacy groups.

## The Transformation of Mental Health

Participants were reminded of the dramatic and positive changes in mental health over the past century, as treatment moved away from asylum patients in shackles to the current era when it has been possible to document the effectiveness of psychopharmaceutical agents and other therapies for many mental disorders. This evolution gradually produced a more caring and humanistic approach to mental problems, a focus on individuals, and efforts to understand the factors that contribute both to mental disorders and to mental health. But the transition has not always been smooth and the results have often been uneven.

While the federally funded community mental health centers, which lasted about two decades, removed patients from large state institutions, countless patients were left without treatment when the federal government returned responsibility for mental health services to the states. For historic reasons, mental health services never received the same insurance coverage as other health care services. These gaps in coverage have limited the availability of treatment for many who needed it.

Ironically, current consumer efforts to gain parity in coverage come at a time when insurers, intent upon limiting services to control costs, have turned to managed care. Though mental illness accounts for 15 percent of health care costs, the percentage of health care dollars now going to provide mental health services has dropped from 8 to 4 percent. Too, since only one practitioner per day can be reimbursed under most plans, the multidisciplinary team approach to mental health care, which had proven effective, has been largely abandoned.

Attitudes toward mental illness have changed markedly in recent years, due primarily to the efforts of consumer advocates who have pushed the mental health research agenda. The willingness of celebrities to talk openly about their own mental disorders and substance abuse problems has reduced stigma. Research for mental health, which 15 years ago ranked tenth on the nation's list of health research priorities, now ranks second.

**Research Advances**

Already, this investment has produced rich dividends and promises to continue to do so. Participants were reminded that recent research has led to greater understanding of how the brain works, including the discovery of functional differences between the two hemispheres. Also, research has uncovered literally dozens of neurotransmitters and neuromodulators and led to development in technology such as PET scans and MRIs capable of measuring what happens in the living brain. There is new understanding of the mechanisms of memory and evidence that the developing brain is molded by experience and that the remodeling process continues throughout life.

In this era, too, diagnosis and classification became more precise, and therapies were tested and validated rigorously in clinical trials. These results were often translated into manuals so that proven techniques could be widely used. Despite concerns that individual and cultural differences might be lost with manualized approaches, the development came at a time when consumers and insurers alike were demanding that health care treatment of all kinds be effective and based on scientific evidence.

Despite the abundant progress, participants were reminded of the problems confronting the field. For example, without accurate information on changing trends in mental health needs, it is impossible to predict what preventive, treatment or rehabilitative services will be needed, or, for that matter, how many and what kinds of providers will be needed or how they should be trained.

**Manpower Needs**

Even without this precise information, though, participants concurred that the mental health professions face a manpower crisis. Child psychiatry provides an extreme example. Currently the field has some 6,000 practitioners with an estimated need of 38,000, and training programs have been unable to attract more residents. Long years of residency and low potential reimbursement rates no doubt contribute. One participant noted that this is one subspecialty where one earns less with more training.

Participants also cited the need to attract more medical students to general psychiatry, to geriatric psychiatry, and to both biological and clinical research in psychiatry. They also urged that pediatricians, family practitioners and other primary care physicians receive more training in mental illness. They especially emphasized the need to increase the number of minority students, not only in medical specialties but also in all of the mental health and related professions.

Psychiatry is not alone, for considerable manpower shortages are found throughout mental health. The number of psychiatric nurses is declining, for instance, as older nurses retire and positions cannot be replaced because of low pay, poor working conditions and new options in nursing careers. Although the public schools provide between 20 and 80 percent of mental health services for children, the current cadre of 31,000 school counselors does not begin to meet the need.

## Training Concerns

Beyond the problem of numbers, participants were concerned about what and how students learn. Though the advent of evidence-based treatment ought to produce more confidence in treatment, some participants worried that too often therapy is still a "black box," offering little certainty about the quality of providers or what they are providing. Issues and new standards for licensure and accreditation both in psychotherapy and psychopharmacology should be addressed. In psychiatry, for instance, mentors in residency programs have varying experience with evidence-based manualized therapies.

A parallel concern was that family practitioners and other physicians, often the first to see patients with mental disorders, need more training in order to diagnose these problems, recognize when to refer for specialized treatment and make appropriate use of psychopharmacological agents. Though social workers and psychologists provide most mental health care, their training, too, needs to be reviewed to be sure these practitioners are aware of evidence-based and manualized therapies and the existence of treatment guidelines.

Participants saw a need for multidisciplinary training and development of a core curriculum identifying the basic knowledge, skills and attitudes needed so providers at all levels will understand about the diagnosis and care of common psychiatric illness. This multidisciplinary effort should not be limited to mental health professionals—the front line psychiatrists, psychologists, social workers, psychiatric nurses and school counselors— but should be expanded to include teachers, ministers, police, parole officers and others who frequently are the first to encounter those with mental health problems.

## Recurring Themes

Certain themes—some not directly related to the education focus of the conference—threaded through the discussions, providing a constant reminder of the complex issues confronting mental health. One involved the crippling impact of inadequate funding, the considerable personal and societal costs of not addressing mental health needs, and the ironic twist that research funding has reached historic levels at a time when the ability to use that research is hindered by lack of funding for clinical care.

Another concerned the context of treatment. Treatment cannot be limited to the individual, participants emphasized. In particular, no child should ever be treated without treating the family, just as no adults should be without attention to children and other members of the family. Also, it is important to take into account the different problems confronting high and low income communities, to appreciate how poverty affects mental health and to consider the contributions of such factors as crime, pollution, racism, environment, and education to both mental health and mental illness.

Turf and guild issues need to be overcome, participants emphasized. This is particularly true of psychiatry that, as a field, has been reluctant to recognize that other professionals are needed to provide valuable mental health care and services. The importance of interdisciplinary staffing of programs should be emphasized and collaboration across the service systems should be fostered.

Also, the mental health professions must pay greater attention to racial, cultural and ethnic differences and to understanding that minority communities are not homogenous. Participants also cited the need throughout health care to increase the pool of students and practitioners from diverse backgrounds and to help all clinicians understand and be more sensitive to the role of cultural differences and their contribution to health and illness.

## Conclusions

The timeliness and critical importance of the goal of enhancing the quality, supply and the diversity of the professional mental health workforce to meet new needs and to function in some new roles was affirmed unanimously. "We have the opportunity and the responsibility to redesign the way we train our future health professionals," one participant commented. Participants emphasized a number of essential core elements, among them mastering new evidence-based therapies; developing the attitudes and learning the skills for teamwork and collaboration across systems; recruitment of minority trainees; teaching respect for and knowledge of diverse cultural values; encouraging rigorous service research; and educating the public, consumer advocacy groups and policy makers about the availability and quality of mental health services.

Therefore, participants concluded that responsibility for implementing their recommendations rests with a wide spectrum of groups, agencies and individuals, including—but not limited to—academic health centers and training programs, professional organizations and societies, consumer advocacy and community groups, credentialing and licensing bodies, and the many local, state, and federal agencies concerned with the mental health of both individuals and communities.

They also recognized that carrying out this responsibility demands new working interfaces and collaboration among systems that currently operate alone. To create this new environment, they urged all parties to work together to identify and eliminate the full range of economic, institutional and "guild" barriers to achieving the goals implicit in the following recommendations.

## Recommendations:

1. *Interdisciplinary Training and Collaboration:*
   **It is now clear that mental health services are best and most efficiently provided by an interdisciplinary team with a common, broad knowledge base. Therefore, all training should:**
   - include specific training curricula on the theory and skills of interdisciplinary collaboration;
   - create models of interdisciplinary treatment in clinical or practicum exercises;

- develop joint programs across disciplines to provide interdisciplinary training to collaborating students;
- identify and reward faculty role models who participate in interdisciplinary professional education and patient care;
- utilize clinical settings that offer strong opportunities for teaching interdisciplinary care;
- and in all cases stress that the success of the collaboration will depend on mutual trust, respect and appreciation of each other's knowledge and skills to best benefit the patient.

2. ***Evidence-based treatments*** **should be taught in all professional schools.**

   For quality assurance, the mastery should be judged by performance criteria, not just the hours spent in taking the courses.

3. ***Recruitment—*** **Given the existing shortage of professionals, an aggressive recruitment program must be developed to attract and train professionals in all the mental health disciplines.**

   Particular emphasis must be placed on broadening representation from diverse racial, ethnic and cultural groups to serve their unmet needs. In addition, because the need is particularly acute, special effort must be given to recruiting and training more child and adolescent psychiatrists and other child mental health professionals.

4. ***A common core curriculum*** **of mental health knowledge, skills and attitudes must be developed.**

   This core curriculum should be taught across all medical specialties and to other mental health professionals to provide both a common vocabulary and an updated knowledge base among those who care for individuals and families. In addition to the formal teaching this core curriculum could be offered, updated and maintained as an Internet-based teaching module.

5. ***Community mental health*** **must be revitalized by removing institutional barriers and developing stronger links across different systems, such as the public welfare, education and justice systems.**

   Workers in those systems should be able to recognize mental illness and be able to identify the appropriate channels to provide care. A core curriculum of key concepts and skills in collaboration should be taught to this workforce.

6. ***Public education*** **about the signs and symptoms and availability of effective treatment for mental disorders, as well as about the social costs incurred by not treating these disorders, is an important means of removing a significant barrier to the appropriate use of mental health services.**

   For the general public, key concepts, as appropriate to all ages, cultural, ethnic/racial, and regional settings, should be provided on the Internet, possibly endorsed and maintained by NIMH, so that all Americans have access to reliable information about the diagnosis and treatment of common mental illnesses. Consumer advocacy groups and the media can be enlisted in public information programs.

7. ***The prevention and treatment of mental health conditions*** **must include not only the individual but also the family and the community.**

   Prevention and treatment must be tailored to specific demographic, socio-cultural, age, gender and ethnic contexts. Families and therapists must all be aware of the significance of these factors as related to a mental disorder.

8. ***Credentialing and licensure.*** **Accreditation requirements and testing should include competence in the areas of collaboration, respect and understanding of diverse cultures, and mastery of all evidence-based therapies, including emphasis on the psychodynamic and cognitive.**

   Whenever possible, officials will judge results using performance-based criteria rather than relying on the number of days or hours spent in didactic sessions. For example, documented reports of actual trainee time spent in interdisciplinary contexts should be included.

# Participants at the Conference

**Beatrix Hamburg, M.D.**
Cornell University Medical College
*Chair*

---

**Sigurd H. Ackerman, M.D.**
St. Luke's-Roosevelt Hospital Center

**Renato D. Alarcon, M.D., M.P.H.**
Emory University

**Paula G. Allen-Meares, Ph.D.**
University of Michigan

**Carole Anderson Ph.D., R.N., F.A.A.N.***
The Ohio State University

**Andrea G. Barthwell, M.D.**
American Society of Addiction Medicine

**Dan G. Blazer, M.D., Ph.D.**
Duke University Medical Center

**Joseph T. Coyle, M.D.**
Harvard Medical School

**Kevin P. Dwyer, M.A., N.C.S.P.***
National Mental Health Association

**Carola Eisenberg, M.D.***
Harvard Medical School

**Glen R. Elliott, Ph.D., M.D.**
University of California - San Francisco

**Vanessa Northington Gamble, M.D., Ph.D.**
Association of American Medical Colleges

**Howard H. Goldman, M.D., Ph.D**
University of Maryland

**Edward M. Hundert, M.D.**
University of Rochester

**James Hudziak, M.D.***
University of Vermont

**Steven E. Hyman, M.D.**
Director, National Institute of Mental Health

**James S. Jackson, Ph.D.**
University of Michigan

**Sherman A. James, Ph.D.**
University of Michigan

**Wynne S. Korr, Ph.D.***
University of California - Berkeley

**Aaron Lazare, M.D.**
University of Massachusetts - Worcester

**David Lewis, M.D.***
Brown University

**Mack Lipkin, Jr., M.D.**
New York University

**Laura F. McNicholas, M.D., Ph.D.**
VA Medical Center/University of Pennsylvania

**Kathleen Merikangas, Ph.D.***
National Institute of Mental Health

**Steven M. Mirin, M.D.**
American Psychiatric Association

**Marian Osterweis, Ph.D.**
Association of Academic Health Centers

**Herbert Pardes, M.D.**
Columbia University

**David J. Sanchez, Jr., Ph.D.**
University of California - San Francisco

**William C. Sanderson, Ph.D.**
Rutgers, The State University of New Jersey

**Rosemary A. Stevens, Ph.D.***
University of Pennsylvania

**Myrna M. Weissman, Ph.D.**
Columbia University

**Ms. Marleen Wong**
Los Angeles Unified School District

**Barry S. Zuckerman, M.D.**
Boston University

**MACY FOUNDATON**

**June E. Osborn, M.D.**

**Martha Wolfgang**

**Tanya Tyler**

**Tashi Dakar Ridley**

**Mary Hager**

* Planning Committee

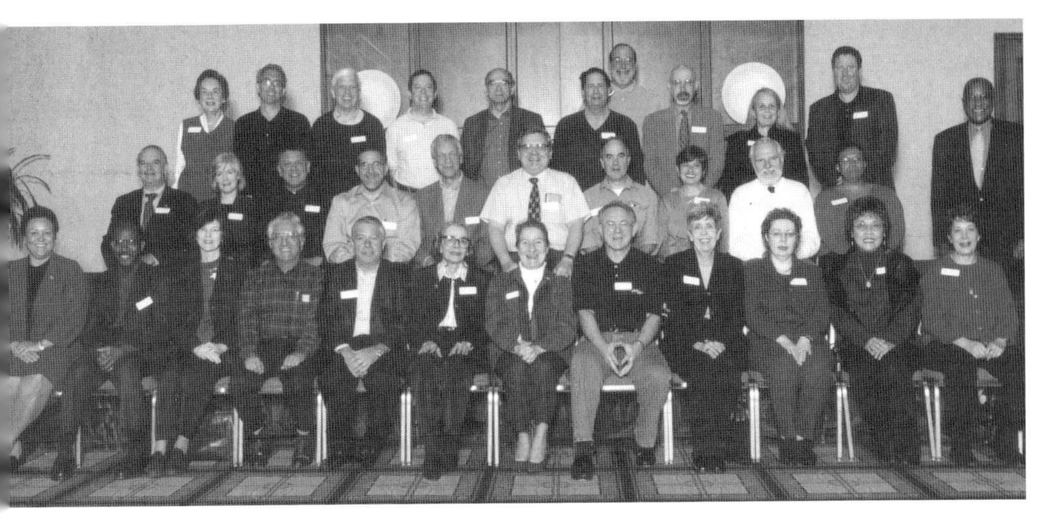

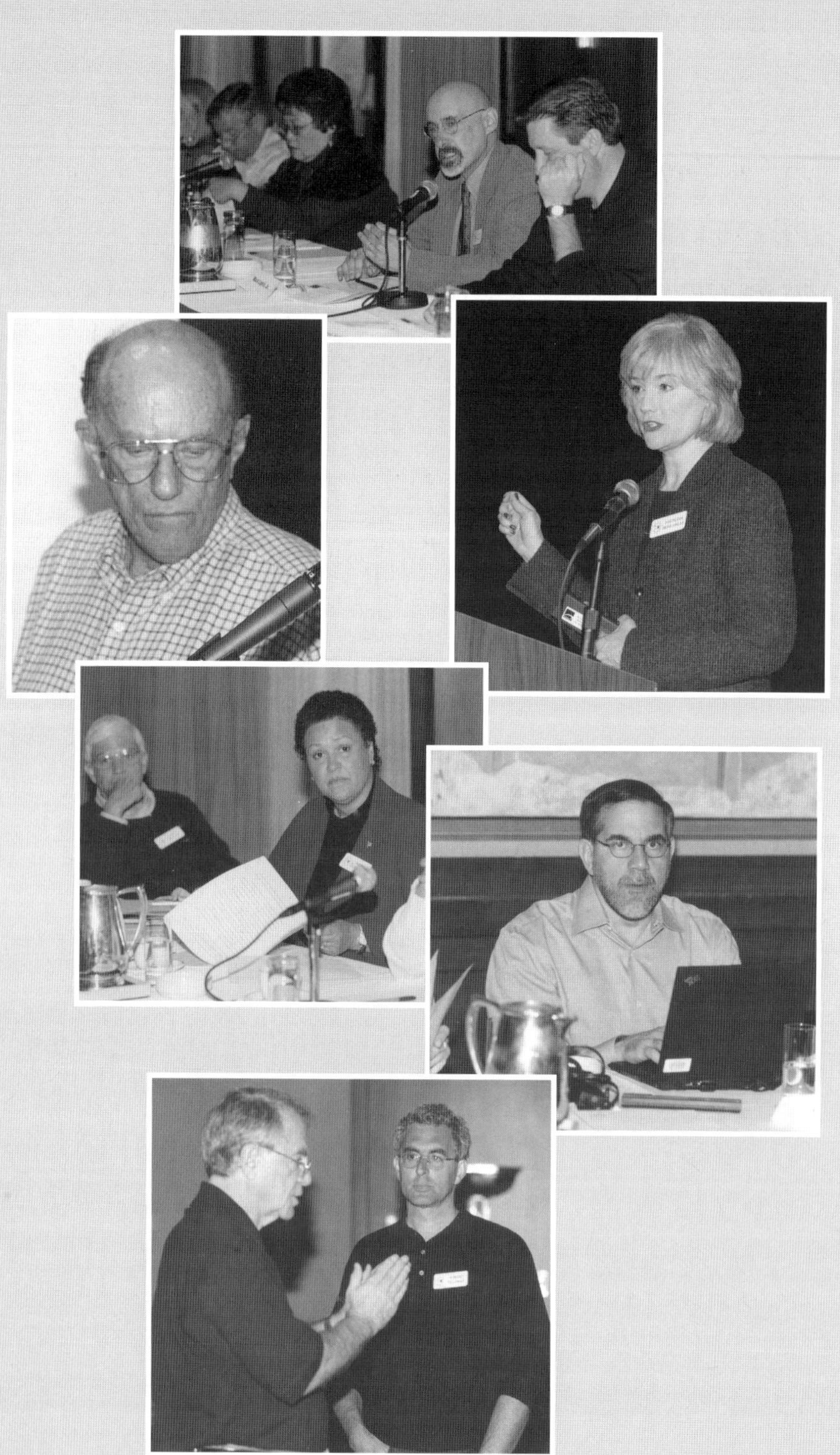

# Session I

## Where Have We Come From, Where Are We Now, Where Are We Headed

*This session provided the conference participants with state of the art reference materials in areas basic to modern psychiatry to serve as a core shared information base for the diverse array of mental health professionals. In this way a context was provided for group members. They could build on this to enrich the discussion by adding their specialized knowledge, experience and perspectives throughout the conference seeking to identify and address the major opportunities and impediments in achieving timely, appropriate education and training of current and future mental health professionals*

# Themes in Twentieth Century American Psychiatry

**Leon Eisenberg, MD**
**Maude and Lillian Presley Professor of Social Medicine and Professor of Psychiatry, Emeritus, Harvard Medical School**

**A Plea for Compassion**

If even skeptical physicists have been shaken up by data from Quasars suggesting that the "fine-structure" constant (an amalgam of the speed of light, the charge of the electron, and the quantum mechanical number known as Planck's constant) has changed by 0.001% since the Big Bang (Seife 2001; Adam 2001), then surely psychiatrists must be cut some slack in view of the tectonic shifts in our field!

## Introduction

As the 19th century ended, psychiatric patients and the doctors who took care of them remained isolated in remote asylums and stigmatized by the fear and shame the patients (and their doctors) aroused. The advances in basic science which had so successfully identified the pathophysiology of medical and surgical diseases had failed wretchedly with mental disorders. They were variously attributed to hereditary degeneration, cerebral asthenia caused by indulgence in masturbation, intestinal intoxication, and other equally unpalatable hypotheses. Psychiatrists managed asylums for the insane, institutions situated at a considerable distance from centers of learning and lacking a research tradition. American asylum psychiatrists, at their 50th Annual Meeting in 1894, were castigated by S. Weir Mitchell (1984), Professor of Neurology at the University of Pennsylvania, in these terms. "Want of competent original work is to my mind the worst symptom of torpor the asylums now present…Where…are your careful scientific reports?…You live alone, uncriticized, unquestioned, out of the healthy conflicts and honest rivalries which keep us [neurologists] up to the mark of the fullest possible competence…"

Whether or not Mitchell's celebration of neurologists was warranted, his criticism of psychiatry certainly was. Only at the turn of the century were the foundations for a research enterprise in psychiatry established – at the New York Pathological Institute (1896), the Psychopathic Hospitals in Ann Arbor (1906) and Boston (1912), and the Henry Phipps Psychiatric Clinic in Baltimore (1913). However, they remained widely-spaced oases in an academic desert. As late as 1958, most US medical schools had at best a part-time psychiatric faculty, constantly hectored as barely discriminable from its clientele and heavily dependent on private practice (Appel and Pearson 1959). At the end of the 20th century, every US medical school has an academic department of psychiatry. Research, basic and clinical, have burgeoned. There has been a veritable revolution in therapeutics. Stigma, still a problem, has diminished. Mental patients are no longer warehoused in large asylums.

What accounts for these very considerable gains, for the problems that persist, and for the new ones that have arisen? In reporting on the evolution of our field during the 20th century, I will proceed from **Concepts** (psychoanalysis; the brain as the organ of the mind; inheritance and genetics; the population sciences); to **Events** (World Wars I and II and Vietnam); to **Venues for Care** (public and private hospital and community services); and finally to **Economic Determinants** (rising costs and imposition of cost controls).

## CONCEPTS

### Psychoanalysis: The Psychogenesis of Mental Disorders

At the turn of the century, within the 10 year period from 1895 when *Studies in Hysteria* (with Breuer) first appeared, to 1901 when *The Interpretation of Dreams* and *The Psychopathology of Everyday Life* were published, to 1905 when *Three Essays on the Theory of Sexuality* was completed, Sigmund Freud created the theory and the practice of psychoanalysis. The late 19th century had been a time of great ferment in psychology: Charcot's theory of hysteria as spontaneous hypnotic states (arising from constitutional weakness of the central nervous system), Bernheim's counter-formulation that hypnotism was but a special instance of general human suggestibility, Janet's concept of dissociated states, Bleuler and Jung's studies of free associations and complexes. Freud was influenced by their work, but it was he whose narrative of psychosexual development, whose metaphorical psychic structures, and whose concept of transference profoundly influenced psychiatry, particularly American psychiatry.

Whether or not psychoanalysis is a "science" and whether or not it is effective as a therapy (a century after its introduction empirical validation is still missing), it has had a powerful impact on psychiatry. Psychoanalytic theory provided plausible explanations for the bizarre symptoms patients exhibited rather than simply categorizing symptoms as disease phenomena. It taught trainees to listen to patients and to try to understand their distress, not simply to classify their diseases or sedate them or lock them away. It highlighted the importance of memory, its vulnerability to distortion, and its centrality to patients' life narratives, the stories we tell ourselves and others. It made clear how those narratives can be self-defeating and defined the task of therapy as helping patients to reconstruct their autobiographies to permit growth. Psychoanalysis helped psychiatry preserve an abiding interest in the individuality of patients while other medical specialists were losing sight of the patient in their preoccupation with the biology of the disease.

The very complexity and counter-intuitiveness of the theory enhanced its allure. It connected the symptoms of mental illness to the psychopathology of everyday life. Psychiatrists learned to help patients by paying attention to their mental symptoms in an era when psychiatry had no "procedures." Although Freud saw no role for psychoanalysis in the treatment of the psychoses, his method inaugurated outpatient psychiatric practice with neurotic patients. Diagnosis and classification — the hallmarks of the medical approach — became increasingly irrelevant to clinical practice; analytically oriented psychotherapy dealt with individual and family dynamics, rather than with syndromes or diseases.

Psychoanalysis only gradually gained a foothold in the U.S.; its influence grew apace with the European intellectual migration after the Nazi *putsch* in Germany. When psychoanalysis was banned from the Congress of Psychology at Munich as "a Jewish science" in October 1933, psychoanalysts in Berlin and Vienna began to leave for the U.K. and the U.S. Jahoda (1969) has estimated that some 100 to 200 European analysts and some 30 to 50 analytically orientated psychologists emigrated to America in the 1930's. That number may seem small, but the membership of the American Psychoanalytic Association was only 135 in 1936 and 249 in 1944 (Canty B: personal communication). The European influx was as significant intellectually as it was numerically; many of the refugees enriched post-Freudian psychoanalytic theory and became leaders in the movement. Psychoanalysis became the dominant trend in academic psychiatry in the U.S. By the early 1960's, although only 10% of American psychiatrists were analysts, more than half of the chairs of medical school departments held membership in psychoanalytic societies (APA 1962). America, in Jahoda's words, became "the world center for psychoanalysis." In contrast, Professor Aubrey Lewis (1953) of the Maudsley noted that "none of the recognized teachers of psychiatry in the undergraduate medical schools of London is a member of the Psychoanalytical Society."

How did psychoanalysis come to be so dominant? There was no other psychological theory that provided as comprehensive an account of the origins of psychopathology. The brain sciences were largely irrelevant to clinical practice. At mid-century, descriptive psychiatrists were held in little esteem because diagnosis was unreliable and made little difference for treatment. The psychiatric pharmacopeia was limited to hypnotics and sedatives. Lack of empirical evidence was not unique to psychiatry. Treatments in all of medicine were based on the authority of "clinical experience." New treatments were assessed by the results reported "by senior members of the medical profession, who had tried them out on a series of patients...and concluded that the outcome was better than that reported by others or by themselves in the past" (Doll 1991). The influence of the authority of one's teachers, the experience of seeing patients improve during psychotherapy (most non-psychotic patients did), the "logic" of psychodynamic explanations and the readiness with which patients desperate for a way out of their dilemmas accepted those explanations combined to make believers of all but the most skeptical of trainees. Those who were non-believers were easily dismissed with *ad hominem* attacks on their unanalyzed "resistance."

**The first double-blind randomized controlled trial (RCT) in medicine**, the United Kingdom Medical Research Council trial of streptomycin for the treatment of tuberculosis, was not carried out until 1949. The RCT rapidly became the gold standard for research in psychopharmacology, but attitudes toward other treatments, notably psychotherapy, were governed by the training physicians had received; research data were yet to come. That this is not a phenomenon limited to psychiatry or to the past is evident from the underuse of evidence-based treatments in current medical practice (Cohen 2001; Euroaspire II 2001).

There was in the '50's and '60's a two-class system of psychiatric care in the U.S. Middle and upper class patients (those who could pay out of pocket and those with generous insurance coverage) sought psychoanalytically oriented out-patient psychotherapy with private practitioners or university staff. Rogow (1970) surveyed a sample of psychoanalysts about the patients they had in treatment.

Not only were they middle or upper class, but not one was Hispanic and very few were black. That was no surprise; the yearly cost of an analysis was more than 80% of the median income of an American worker. Psychiatric trainees vied for opportunities to treat young, articulate, and well-educated patients with anxiety disorders. Lower class patients with psychoses were "cared for" in grossly under-resourced state or county mental hospitals. Although there were dedicated psychiatrists in the public sector, all too many were foreign-trained and worked in the state hospitals because they had no choice; they needed to qualify for licensure; their psychiatric training was marginal; they had limited command of English. The paradox that the most seriously ill patients received care from the least well-trained psychiatrists did not escape the attention of the National Association for the Mentally Ill; it remains militant in demanding that public funding for service and research focus on the seriously and chronically ill. Its members hail biological psychiatry; dispute the claims for care of non-psychotic patients; and doubt the value of psychotherapy. They have not forgotten psychiatry's role in blaming parents as pathogenic agents in schizophrenia.

In 1962, I had described my dismay that "in some centers…almost all the residents enter personal analysis…in my observation, it has been the bright and not the incompetent, the curious and not the unimaginative residents who have been attracted to psychoanalysis and thus lost to research, university teaching and public service" (Eisenberg 1962). My dismay stemmed from (a) restrictions on the resident's geographic mobility for the duration of a didactic analysis which might last for five to seven years, (b) the press to earn supplementary income from after hours private practice to pay for the analysis, (c) the acquisition of a therapeutic technique altogether inappropriate to meet public need, and (d) lack of curiosity because they thought they possessed the exclusive road to salvation. But they did listen to patients and try to understand them, albeit with "the third ear" and through arcane symbols and metaphors.

Forty years later, the pendulum has swung so far in the other direction that young psychiatrists may no longer be listening to patients with any ear. Physician applicants to teaching institutes affiliated with the American Psychoanalytic Association numbered 265 in 1977; they fell to 109 in 1987 and to 88 in 1996 (Myrna Weissman and Joan Abramowitz, personal communication). The institutes do not suffer from a dearth of students; the number of non-physician applicants has risen steadily since the 1986 federal court decision that non-physicians could not be excluded from analytic training programs because such exclusions would constitute restraint of trade. What explains the decline in medical candidates? In part, it stems from the greater allure of competing career lines in psychopharmacology and neuroscience; in part, the reason is economic: medical students graduate with far greater indebtedness than was the case a generation ago when many could afford to undertake a didactic analysis. According to AAMC data, 81% of graduating US students have educational debts averaging $95,000. Cost is now a deterrent in view of the debt to be repaid. Empirical research in psychotherapy never did have much cachet in departments of psychiatry; it has become the province of departments of psychology. It is a rare psychiatrist who opts for a research career in psychotherapy. Indeed, few opt for research careers at all!

## The Evaluation of the Psychotherapies

Through the '50s, '60s and '70s, there was a large psychotherapy sector untroubled by the lack of evidence for effectiveness; the Scots' verdict of "unproven" effectiveness had no impact on training or practice. The flavor of the times can best be conveyed by waggish comments from cynics. At the 1952 American Psychological Association Conference on Graduate Education in Clinical Psychology, Morris Parloff of NIH commented: "Therapy is an undefined technique which is applied to unspecified problems with non-predictable outcome. For this technique, we recommend rigorous training." Paul Meehl (1965) offered a tongue-in-cheek rationale for the difficulty in demonstrating effectiveness. He estimated that three out of four patients would either recover on their own or remain ill, whether or not they received psychotherapy and that only one in four therapists had the skill to make a difference for the potentially responsive patients. Thus, "if ? represents the upper bound on the proportion of patients…who are appropriate and let ? also represent an upper bound on therapists who are good at their job…the joint probability of a suitable patient getting to a suitable therapist is about 0.06, a very small tail to wag the statistical dog in an outcome study."

One of the few serious students of psychotherapy, Jerome Frank (1961), compared research in the field to:

> "the nightmarish game of croquet in *Alice and Wonderland* in which the mallets were flamingos, the balls hedgehogs, and the wickets soldiers. Since the flamingo would not keep its head down, the hedgehogs kept unrolling themselves and

> the soldiers were always wandering to other parts of the field…it was a very difficult game indeed."

Frank recognized that psychotherapy outcomes were better than wait-list comparison groups but remarkably similar to one another despite differences in the theories and techniques to which therapists professed allegiance. He concluded that a number of non-specific psychological processes were common to successful psychotherapy: an intense confiding relationship with a therapist; a set of "explanations" for the patient's distress; suggested alternative ways of dealing with the identified problems; the arousal of hope; and the restoration of morale. His conclusion offended proponents of all the schools of psychotherapy. Two decades later, Smith, Glass, and Miller (1980) made a more successful foray when they reported the results of meta-analysis of extant studies of psychotherapy. Their book was widely hailed by practitioners as establishing the effectiveness of psychotherapy because most treatments had a significant effect size; however, once again, outcome differences between treatments or between novices and experts was hard to detect.

Myrna Weissman's (2001) paper on the "Paradox of psychotherapy" and her background paper for this Macy Conference provides an elegant analysis of the development and present status of Evidence Based (psycho)Therapies (EBT). The matter will not be pursued further here except to note the irony that just as EBT has proved its worth, the economics of managed care has sharply restricted the ability of practitioners to provide psychotherapy!

Until recently there was no formal requirement that psychiatric residents learn about (let alone acquire competence in) alternate forms of psychotherapy. To the extent psychotherapy is taught at present (rather than being swamped by psychopharmacology), it remains mostly psychodynamic (that is, based on psychoanalytic principles) reflecting the training of the senior teachers in academic programs (Luhrmann 2000). The Accreditation Council for Graduate Medical Education in January 2001 published (*http://www.acgme.org/req/400pr101.asp*) new program requirements for residency training in psychiatry. Those requirements include (VI. B. 2): "The program must demonstrate that residents have acquired competency in at least the following forms of treatment: (a) brief therapy (b) cognitive-behavior therapy (c) combined psychotherapy and psychopharmacology (d) psychodynamic therapy and (e) supportive therapy." To address the challenge of measuring competence, the American Association of Directors of Psychiatry Residency Training has established a task force (with assistance from experts in each modality of psychotherapy) to operationalize these competencies in order to assess residents' performance and to plan for remediation if they fall short (Lisa Mellman, personal communication). The decision to evaluate education by measuring competencies rather than by number of seminars attended, number of patients seen and years of training is a major positive change. Psychiatry for once is leading the way.

## The Brain as the Organ of the Mind

In the last half of the 19th Century, progress in pathology and bacteriology uncovered the pathogenesis of many diseases; it had revealed disappointingly little about mental disorders. Thus, it was a major event in 1913 when Noguchi and Moore found *Treponema pallidum* in the brain of patients with general paresis, just eight years after Schaudinn and Hoffman identified the spirochete as the cause of syphilis. General paresis was an appealing model for the pathogenesis of psychosis. In its early stages, it could mimic any psychiatric disorder. Success in unraveling its pathogenesis as a manifestation of tertiary syphilis appeared to presage similar discoveries for the other psychoses. The long and hitherto fruitless search for brain pathology appeared to be over; the discovery of the spirochete in the brain was seen as the rebirth of neuropathology.

To the distress of neuropsychiatrists, dementia praecox and manic depressive psychosis continued to be impervious to laboratory research. Report after report of the discovery of histologic lesions in the brain proved to be due to artifacts. Neurochemistry was unsuccessful in manipulating brain cerebrosides and other insoluble tissue components. The failure of available methods to reveal pathologic changes in the brain in schizophrenia and manic depressive disease crystallized a belief that they were psychogenic.[1]

During the 1950's and '60's, when clinical psychiatry in the United States enjoyed a considerable expansion in faculty representation, in time in the medical curriculum, and in recruits to its ranks (Webster 1969), its methods were primarily psychological; its departments were staffed by clinicians; training emphasized the meaning of the present illness in the context of the patient's past and the therapeutic use of the doctor patient relationship. Psychiatry became particularly attractive to the clinically oriented medical student who found it one of the few specialties with a persisting concern for the patient as a person in an era of organ-centered medicine.[2] General practice, which might have provided an alternative, had almost ceased to enlist further recruits in the U.S. because of its low prestige, difficult working conditions, and isolation from the medical mainstream.

So matters stood until the care of patients with psychotic disorders was radically changed by a series of chance discoveries: of reserpine's psychotropic effects when it was used to treat hypertension; of chlorpromazine as a "tranquilizer" during research on anesthesia; of iproniazid as a euphoriant when it was used to treat tuberculosis; of the anti-depressant properties of imipramine in therapeutic trials for neuroleptic effects (Kuhn 1958); and of the anti-manic effects of lithium when Cade (1949) found that the lithium urate (chosen solely because of the solubility of the compound in urine) caused sedation in guinea pigs. The serendipity of these findings does not minimize their importance but it does emphasize the lack of coherent biological theories to guide their discovery; those theories emerged *post hoc* in the effort to account for the empirical findings.

The new therapeutic armamentarium had major consequences for the practice of psychiatry. It provided means for aborting acute psychotic episodes and for minimizing recurrences. Because remissions could be induced in a relatively short time frame (and because insurance coverage became available), psychiatric units in general hospitals expanded rapidly. Because the new agents were thought to be relatively syndrome specific, diagnosis and classification now became important clinical issues for effective patient care and paved the way for DSM-III and DSM-IV (for better or for worse).[3] Not the least of the benefits of psychopharmacology was the development of methodologies for the double-blind evaluation of the new therapeutic agents, drugs, social interventions and psychotherapies (Klerman 1974). The discovery of psychotropic drugs stimulated the development of the neurosciences, which have flowered in an extraordinary fashion.[4]

The scientific yield has been extraordinary. A half century ago norepinephrine and acetylcholine were the only neurotransmitters known; their receptors had not yet been identified. The brain was viewed as an telephone switchboard with its connections precisely wired according to genetic instructions. Today candidate neurotransmitters near 100 and still counting; the identification of cell surface receptors grows apace. We now know of neuromodulators, intercellular chemical messengers which bias the responsiveness of synaptic elements. In effect, the brain modifies its own response to incoming stimuli.

The plasticity of brain structure is evident from the discovery of competition between axon terminals which proliferate in excess during early development. Activity determines survivorship. It is now possible to examine the molecular concomitants of learning and to distinguish the chemical events underlying short-term versus long-term memory. The more we learn about the complex interaction between the components of the brain as shaped by its environment, the less tenable is a purely internalist account of brain function. Who would have believed that glial cells, dismissed as the "glue" that held the brain together, might have a role in information processing in the brain (Kast 2001)?

The great Ramon y Cajal had declared in 1913 that nerve paths in adult brain are "fixed, ended, immutable. Everything may die, nothing may be regenerated." So I was taught; so I believed. Research has now unearthed an unrecognized potential for producing new neurons in the mammalian central nervous system (Johansson 1999). Progenitor cells within the dentate gyrus of the hippocampus continue to produce new granule cells throughout life in human brains (Erikson *et al.* 1998). Granule cell proliferation is diminished by stress (Gould *et al.* 1998, 1999) and enhanced by environmental enrichment even in aging animals (Kempermann *et al.* 1998). Not only is a developing brain molded by experience but the process continues throughout life. Finger representation in the cortex is larger on the right in professional violinists (in response to the hand fingering the strings) and it is larger than it is in non-musicians (Elbert *et al.* 1995). Finger representation is enlarged in Braille readers (Sterr *et al.* 1998) and sensory expression shrinks after deafferentation. Brain function and structure are constantly in flux. Indeed, it was recently reported that finger representation in the cortex of a patient with severed hands shrank post injury, but following successful replacement of the hand, the cortical area re-expanded!

The success of neuroscience has exacted costs. The very elegance of research in neuroscience has led psychiatry to focus so exclusively on the brain as an organ that the experience of the patient as a person has receded below the horizon of our vision. We had for so long been pilloried by our medical and surgical colleagues as witch-doctors and wooly-minded thinkers that we now seek professional respectability by adhering to a reductionistic model of mental disorder. We have traded the one-sidedness of the "brainless" psychiatry of the first half of the 20th century for a "mindless" psychiatry of the second half (Eisenberg 1986). Even psychoanalysts have found it convenient to recall that Freud (1914), himself a product of 19th century reductionism, cautioned his followers that "all our provisional ideas will some day be based on an organic substructure...we take this possibility into account when we substitute special forces in the mind for special chemical substances."

## Inheritance and Genetics

Fifty years ago genetics was anathema in psychiatry. Now it is all the rage. The pendulum has swung from "it's all nurture" to "it's all nature." What accounts for the intellectual tsunami?

It had been known since antiquity that like breeds like and that mental diseases cluster in families, observations compatible with inheritance. What was inherited and how it was inherited remained a mystery. The first real clue, the work of Mendel in the 19th century, was lost in obscure publications and was not to be rediscovered until the turn of the century. Methods of study were statistical; racist assumptions were ubiquitous.

Francis Galton coined the term eugenics: the improvement of the race by selective breeding. Karl Pearson, the bio-statistician who developed the methodology for the correlation coefficient and the chi-square statistic, lamented the "potentially dysgenic effect" of unchecked Jewish immigration from Russia and Poland on the Anglo-Saxon stock of Great Britain (Pearson and Moul 1925). Ernst Rudin, recognized as the founder of psychiatric genetics, argued that homosexuality is a genetically determined "diseased form of degeneracy" in the first volume of the *Archiv fur Rassen und Gesselleschaftsbiologie* in 1904. The same Rudin was a contributor to the Law for the Prevention of Genetically Diseased Offspring passed by the Reichstag in 1933. Eleven years later, he received a medal from the Third Reich as "a pathbreaker in the field of human hereditary care" (Proctor 1988).

The conflation of genetics with Nazi racist ideology thoroughly discredited genetics in the decades after World War II. Eric Stromgren (1994) reports that in the '20's and '30's, most academic and asylum psychiatrists in Europe believed that schizophrenia and manic depressive disorder were inherited; after the war "genetics had become a dirty word." He was unable to discuss with most American psychiatrists even "the possibility of a genetic contribution to etiology." Stromgren ascribed their negative attitudes to their fealty to psychoanalysis; but the aversion to Nazism was far more instrumental.

At mid-century, there was a huge intellectual chasm between hereditarians and environmentalists based on common shared misconceptions. Both sides mistook genes for fate; both believed that "genotype determines phenotype." Environmentalists rejected the therapeutic pessimism implicit in a reductionistic view of genetics. They preferred to view the organism as a *tabula rasa* and sought the psychogenic origins of psychosis. They dismissed Kallmann's (1946) twin studies showing remarkably high (86%) concordance rates in monozygotic (MZ) versus 14% in dizygotic (DZ) twins. Kallmann's work was subjected to unrelenting and justified methodologic criticism; it suffered from ascertainment bias; lack of blinding when co-twins were evaluated; fuzzy diagnostic categories; and the like. But the baby went out with the bathwater. More rigorous studies have found much lower pair-wise MZ concordance rates (30 to 40%) but the MZ/DZ differences are robust enough to demonstrate a role for inheritance (Kringlen 2000). The critics of genetic determinism failed to apply the same methodological scrutiny to their own even woolier hypotheses (the "schizophrenigenic" mother, schizophrenia as the outcome of faulty communication in the family; the schizophrenic patient as a rebel in an insane world, etc.).

What accounts for the resurrection of genetics in psychiatry? It resulted from progress in molecular genetics: defining genes as biological structures, beginning with the Beadle-Tatum 1941 "one gene — one enzyme" hypothesis, Avery's 1944 demonstration that the transforming principle in pneumococcus was DNA, Watson and Crick's identification of the DNA double-helix in 1953, and the progressive refinement of ever more precise laboratory methods, (including restriction fragment length polymorphisms [RFLP's]) to identify the molecular basis of gene mutation.

Fifteen years ago, amidst great controversy, bold proposals were advanced to map the entire human genome by using automated methods for DNA analysis. That project was provisionally "completed" in 2001 by two competing teams, one in the public sector, under the lead of the National Human Genome Research Institute (reported in *Nature* 15 February 2001) and the other in the private sector;

Celera Genomics (reported in *Science* 16 February 2001). Both maps have sizeable gaps; their topographies do not fully correspond. Both lead to estimates of about 30,000 human genes, far fewer than expected. A new estimate, computed by extrapolation from the number of novel genes in non-overlapping areas in the two maps, suggests the total may be closer to 42,000 (Hogenesch et al. 2001). Nonetheless, the accomplishment in mapping the genome is staggering. Some two million single nucleotide polymorphisms have been mapped in the human genome and a public-private consortium has set out to map some 300,000 haplotypes (genetic markers close enough on the chromosome to be inherited together) the new maps will accelerate the process of gene localization.

The outline of the map of the human genome is a major milestone, but there is still a long itinerary from the linear DNA code to the controls on the methylation of DNA, to the translation of RNA into protein, to the folding of that protein into a three dimensional configuration, to the post-translational addition of sugars to the protein backbone, to protein-protein interactions, to inputs from the cellular surround and so on step after step until the phenotype results. These are non-trivial steps. Werner von Heisenberg, the physicist, let it be known in the 1930s that he had put together the broad outlines of a theory unifying gravity and electromagnetism and that he would publish it, once he had sorted out the details. Wolfgang Pauli, a physicist with a biting sense of humor, sent a postcard to a friend. On it he drew a frame around a blank space. His message read: "This is to show that I can paint like Titian. Only the details are missing" (Lindley 2001). Filling in those "details" will occupy geneticists and developmentalists for decades to come.

Nature and nurture are to phenotype as length and width are to the area of a rectangle. There is no way to assign a percentage of that area to its length and another percentage to its width. Without length and width, there would be no rectangle and no area. In similar terms, every phenotypic trait is the outcome of genes expressed in particular environments. Agreed, there are limiting cases at either extreme; that is, lethal genes incompatible with fetal viability and environments lethal to every genome. When tons of carbon dioxide erupted from the bottom layer of Lake Nyos in the Cameroon on August 21, 1986, the cloud suffocated everything in its path as it rolled down the hill. By next morning, 1700 people and countless animals were dead (Clark 2001). There were no gene-based exceptions. In most circumstances, however, gene effects on the phenotype have been modified by the environments the organism has encountered and phenotypic environmental effects on the phenotype are dependent on the genomes of the organisms on which they have acted. Between genotype and phenotype, there is a long and complex process of interaction within and between cells, between cells and organs, and between organism and environment.[5]

**Population Sciences: Epidemiology and Public Health**

Surveys of mental disorder in the U.S. population date as far back as 1855 (Jarvis 1855/1971). Because they were based on treated prevalence (that is, patients identified because they were registered in a hospital or a clinic), prevalence was always higher in geographic areas with greater service. Further, doubt was cast on the data because of the unreliability of psychiatric diagnoses; clinicians disagreed with each other almost as often as they agreed. One of the first modern community prevalence studies was carried out in the Eastern Health District of Baltimore in the 1950's. About 10% of the non-institutional urban population was found to suffer from a mental illness at a point in time (Pasamanick 1959). A more ambitious attempt, the Midtown Manhattan study, abandoned "diagnosis" and focused on symptoms and disabilities. It reported estimates that 23.4% of persons in the community exhibited impairment because of mental distress and "found" that in some poor minority communities, impairment exceeded 90%, a conclusion absurd on the face of it (Srole *et al.* 1962)!

The issue of diagnostic validity was brought into focus by Mort Kramer (1969) who initiated studies on the puzzling discrepancy between U.S. and U.K. data on the prevalence of schizophrenia and depression (higher rates for schizophrenia and lower rates for depression in the U.S.). NIMH funding enabled panels of U.K. and U.S. psychiatrists to examine a common set of American and British patients (via videotape). The findings were unequivocal; it was not disease prevalence, but disease criteria that differed between the two countries. Once criteria were standardized, the difference largely evaporated. That study gave impetus to the development of standardized psychiatric interviews and led to an operationalized diagnostic manual, DSM III in 1980.

The NIMH underwrote a comprehensive study of the prevalence of mental disorders in the United States employing the new instruments. Populations were sampled in five Epidemiologic Catchment Areas

(New Haven, Baltimore, St. Louis, Durham and Los Angeles). Not only was diagnosable mental disorder found to be common (overall annual prevalence: 20%), but only one in five of those who met criteria for a mental or addictive disorder were actually receiving care (Robins and Regier 1991). The majority of those in need got such care as they received from primary care practitioners rather than from specialist mental health services. Regier and his colleagues (1978) coined the phrase: "the *de facto* U.S. mental health services system" to describe the pattern of care actually available in the community as opposed to the system on paper (Regier *et al.* 1978).

The message was unambiguous: the magnitude of the need for treatment is such that the only possible public health solution is to enhance the capacity of the primary health care system to provide mental health treatment (Eisenberg 1992).[6] Epidemiology had brought home forcefully the dimensions of the problem, dimensions that hospital and clinic based studies could not have revealed (Goldberg and Huxley 1992). Psychiatry has not yet fashioned an adequate response. During the late 70's, when public policy subsidized primary care training, the APA fought to have psychiatry designated a "primary care specialty." That absurd proposal failed. Psychiatrists have yet to make a commitment to improve the skills of family practitioners, to make themselves available as consultants for patients who fail to respond to treatment, and to be responsible for the most difficult cases. The integration of psychiatry and medicine remains to be achieved.

## EVENTS

### World War I

The high rates of psychiatric casualties during prolonged trench warfare and the bizarre symptomatology soldiers exhibited were entirely unexpected by the medical services of either side. Because exposure to intense artillery fire was the most obvious and frightening phenomenon, soldiers called the mental breakdown in combat "shell shock." Initially, some neuropsychiatrists used a similar formulation in attributing the symptoms to blast effects on the brain. This theory had to be abandoned when soldiers remote from an explosion and when soldiers who thought they had been exposed to toxic gases exhibited the same symptoms. "Brain concussion" was replaced by psychological explanations as it was recognized that patients with war neuroses improved more rapidly when they were treated near the front without being evacuated to rear hospitals.[7]

Immediacy of response was crucial; it was essential to establish the expectancy that the soldier would return to his unit. The longer a soldier was away from the front, the more he felt like a coward; to avoid thinking of himself as a coward, he had to think of himself as sick. Recognition of the negative effects of labeling led to the abandonment of the terms "shell shock" and "war neurosis." Casualties were retagged as "not yet diagnosed (nervous)." The soldier was told that a short rest would cure the fatigue and anxiety resulting from stress.

In the war's wake, there were high rates of persistent "war neuroses" among German veterans who received disability pensions for psychiatric symptoms. After World War II, German policy changed and offered pensions only to medical or neurological combat casualties. In parallel (or was it in consequence?), rates of "war neuroses" among German veterans of WW II were far lower than they had been after WW I.

**World War II**

Of some 18 million men screened for the military draft, almost two million were rejected for emotional or mental defect. Another three quarters of a million were prematurely separated from the service for symptoms exhibited during training. During World War I draft rejection rates were at most 2%. Yet rates of breakdown in service were 12% in World War II as against 2% in the first war!

Under combat conditions, the Army Medical Corps relearned the lessons of World War I: the key role of forward treatment for "exhaustion" rather than "neurosis;" the importance of unit morale and group cohesion in maintaining the effectiveness of soldiers and reducing breakdown; inability to screen out inevitable psychiatric casualties; rates depend on unit and combat environment as well as individual susceptibility. Appropriate interventions can return the majority of psychiatric casualties to combat duty" (Jones 2000).

The War had an extraordinary impact on American psychiatry. It initiated the process of revising diagnosis and classification; it resulted in a marked expansion in psychiatric manpower; it fostered federal support for psychiatric research; and, perhaps most important of all, it sparked the development of an exigent approach to care (the open hospital and community based treatment).

First, the Standard Nomenclature of Disease, based on case experience in state mental hospitals and adopted in 1934, proved entirely unsatisfactory for use by psychiatrists in induction stations, in military service, and in the Veterans Administration. The Armed Forces undertook a sweeping revision of the classification in 1945, as did the Veterans Administration; the result was three U.S. systems, none fully compatible with the International Statistical Classification! With support from the NIMH, the American Psychiatric Association prepared its first Diagnostic and Statistical Manual of Mental Disorders (1951) which became the benchmark.

Second, it led to a substantial expansion in psychiatric manpower. Trained psychiatrists were so few in number when WW II began that the Armed Services had to press general physicians into psychiatric duty after short training courses (producing derisively labeled "90 day wonders"). Many of those pressed into duty became so engrossed by their clinical experience that they undertook formal psychiatric training at the War's end. Membership in the American Psychiatric Association, only 2,423 in 1940, more than doubled to 5,856 in 1950; ten years later, it almost doubled again to 11,037.[8]

Third, in the aftermath of a war in which scientific research had played so vital a role in the allied victory, the National Mental Health Act was passed overwhelmingly by the Congress in 1946. The Act gave the new National Institute of Mental Health a mandate to foster psychiatric research.

Fourth, the focus on the situational determinants of breakdown, on the importance of exigent treatment and the need for the rapid reintegration into social roles provided impetus for brief hospitalization, open hospitals, group methods and the community mental health movement.

## The Vietnam War (1961 – 1973; America's longest war)

The most striking psychiatric phenomenon in Vietnam was the low rate of identified psychiatric casualties and the relative absence of combat fatigue. Unique to Vietnam was the inverse relationship between rates of servicemen wounded in action and those who became neuropsychiatric casualties. As the war dragged on, an increasing number of characterological problems surfaced: racial incidents, disciplinary problems, and substance use. Was the low rate of psychiatric casualties related to the high rates of substance use?

Concern about substance abuse among service men in Vietnam

paralleled concern about drug use in the U.S. The availability of cheap heroin ($6 per day to maintain a habit) grown in the golden triangle of Thailand, Burma, and Laos assured easy access. At peak use in October 1971, Robins (1973) estimates that almost half (45%) of Army enlisted men were using narcotics (heroin or opium) and better than 75% marijuana and alcohol. Almost half of narcotic users reported themselves to have been addicted. Yet, on follow-up, Robins found that very few of the identified heroin users continued regular use after demobilization. Most who did had been addicted prior to service. For the others, substance availability, boredom, absence of family and community, and lack of commitment to an unpopular war led to high user rates which abated promptly after leaving Vietnam.

Persistent mental distress after exposure to catastrophic situations is as old as recorded history but the formal identification of what we now know as the Post-Traumatic Stress Syndrome (intrusion of memories of trauma, numbing and avoidance, and hyperarousal to stimuli evoking recollections) only took place in the aftermath of the Vietnam War. PTSD did not appear in the official psychiatric nomenclature until DSM III (1980). A political struggle waged by social workers and activists on behalf of Vietnam veterans who demanded acknowledgement of their distress (Young 1995) was instrumental in legitimating PTSD as a psychiatric diagnosis.

## VENUES OF CARE

### State and County Mental Hospital System

In the first half of the 19th century, asylums for the insane represented progress; they reversed earlier eras of neglect and mistreatment in poorhouses and jails. Asylum superintendents insisted that to achieve therapeutic goals hospitals have no more than 250 beds. As the 19th century drew to a close, hospital size grew steadily despite Adolf Meyer's warning that the "apparent administrative economy" of greater size would "overrule effectiveness of our work against mental disorder" (Grob 1983). The number of in-patients in state and county mental hospitals continued to increase dramatically during the first half of the 20th century: from 188,000 in 1910 to 512,000 in 1950. At that rate of growth, the census was projected to exceed 700,000 within 20 years. Instead, it peaked at 560,000 in 1955, slowly receded in the next two decades (to 535,000 in 1960 and to 338,000 in 1970), and fell precipitously in the last twenty five years.

Through the first 50 years, the mental hospital system functioned to "protect" communities and families from dealing with distressed and often distressing patients. "Economies of scale" rationalized increasing size; the patient's quality of life was not part of the cost-benefit equation. Institutions operated on rigid schedules tailored to bureaucratic needs. Locked doors, loss of personal control, the regimentation of everyday life, separation from family and community, and unoccupied days of hopeless despair led to a "social breakdown syndrome" superimposed on the initial illnesses that led to admission (Gruenberg 1967). The longer the stay, the "sicker" the patient became. The symptoms generated by anomie were attributed to disease in the patient. The hospital contributed to the very chronicity that fed its growth.

Indeed, so grim was the prognosis for chronic mental illness that psychosurgery, a desperate remedy for a desperate condition, was employed in private, public, VA, and university hospitals. Pressman (1999) estimated that between 1936 and 1951, about 20,000 patients underwent prefrontal lobotomies. Psychosurgery was largely abandoned in the 1950's; it was not because of new scientific evidence; there had never been good evidence. The procedure was given up because the newly discovered psychotropic drugs were demonstrably more effective and far less toxic.

Although the psychotropic drugs are commonly credited for the emptying out of state hospitals, that was true only in large, understaffed, and poorly led institutions where patients had been warehoused (Odegaard 1964). The philosophy of the open hospital and the provision of services in the community led to much earlier discharge well before the wide availability of drugs in organized and well managed hospitals (Shepherd *et al.* 1961). However, the effectiveness of psychotropic drugs made it far easier to establish acute psychiatric units in general hospitals and to maintain patients in the community without hospitalization.

Deinstitutionalization was initiated by three factors: a socio-political movement in favor of open hospitals and community mental health services; the advent of psychotropic drugs able to abort psychotic episodes; and a financial imperative to shift costs from state to federal budgets. Failure to track patients after discharge enabled state mental health authorities to declare "victory." There was no tabulation of the tens of thousands of elderly patients who were "transinstitutionalized" from asylums to nursing homes and the thousands of young adult patients who were discharged to homelessness on city streets.

Discharging chronic patients well before aftercare services were provided afforded fiscal relief to the states which had borne the full burden for the mental hospital system. Once patients were discharged, their housing, medical and general welfare costs were jointly shared between federal and state budgets. The passage of Medicaid and Medicare in 1965 was instrumental in shifting the care of elderly persons from mental hospitals to chronic care nursing facilities. The two HHS programs became the largest supporters of the mentally ill in the U.S. without ever being labeled mental health programs. By 1985, nursing homes had more than 600,000 residents diagnosed as mentally ill, largely as the result of Medicaid (Grob 1994).

Budgetary savings lagged well behind discharge rates. Dismantling existing state hospitals was politically contentious. In rural communities, the state hospital might be the major employer. Though services were, in principle, to follow patients back into the community, "chronic" hospital attendants, protected by civil service, were unprepared to become community health workers and unwilling to move to new job sites. In consequence, the inpatient census declined far more rapidly in the first several decades than did the number of state mental hospital employees.

Residential treatment beds in state and county mental hospitals declined from 413,000 to 63,000 between 1970 and 1998. Despite a small increase in beds in private psychiatric hospitals (from 14,000 to 34,000) and in general hospital psychiatric beds (from 22,000 to 54,000), the ratio of hospital and residential treatment beds per 100,000 civilian population declined from 264 to 112. Over that time interval, despite an increase in hospital admissions from 1,300,000 to 2,300,000 (*i.e.* from a rate of 644 to 875 per 100,000). Length of stay fell rapidly and first admissions and repeat admissions and outpatient treatment episodes rose (from about 2 million to 7 million).

For most patients, deinstitutionalization has been an extraordinary benefit, however unsatisfactory aftercare remains. However, many former psychiatric patients were left homeless and without care. With the downsizing of state hospitals, chronic patients are being diverted into jails and prisons (Torrey 1997).

## Costs of Care

The application of science to medicine led to an exponential increase in the capabilities of the health care system to diagnose, treat and prevent disease in the years since World War II. Along with the new knowledge came the growth of medical specialization, an increase in the years of training required to qualify as a specialist, and a vast increase in the number of health care workers needed to support the work of physicians. A ratio of one "para-medical" to one doctor at the beginning of the century had become 10 to 1 by 1970 and 15 to 1 by its end. *Pari passu*, there was an enormous growth in medical care expenditures. The proportion of the gross domestic product consumed by health care rose from about 4% in the 40's to 13% in 1999. Health Care Financing Administration projections anticipate a further increase to 15.9% of GDP by the year 2010! (*http://www.hcfa.gov/stats/NHE_Proj/proj2000/tables/t1.htm*)

When I was a house officer in 1946, no one talked about costs in teaching hospitals. I cannot recall once being asked not to admit, or to discharge a patient early, because of the costs of care. Quite to the opposite! To spare patients' out-of-pocket costs, we admitted them for diagnostic study because insurance perversely covered tests for hospitalized, but not for ambulatory, patients. Why were teaching hospital costs below the radar screen? For one thing, the "hotel" component of hospital costs was low because hospital workers were paid barely subsistence wages. Second, philanthropy met a sizeable portion of expenditures. Third, attending physicians "donated" teaching hours in return for admitting privileges to hospitalize private patients. Fourth, private pavilion charges subsidized ward costs; the Robin Hood principle was widely employed in teaching hospitals until insurers refused to cross-subsidize. Fifth, overhead costs in outpatient dispensaries for "charity" patients were low (hospitals hardly bothered to bill because payment was so unlikely from an uninsured population); hospital managers were few and were paid modest salaries.

House officers were few and paid hardly at all. The total number of interns and residents (all years) across the United States was just under 16,000 in 1945. By the year 2000, the number had grown to 97,000, some 5200 of them psychiatric trainees (Barzansky and Etzel 2001). As an intern in 1946, I received food, a bed in a shared room, hospital whites and $25 a month for a stipend. Costs per house officer in 2001/02 (stipend plus fringe averaged across four years of residency) are now about $50,000 (Boston data). Multiplied by the number of house officers, the total cost is on the order of $4.8 billion.[9]

I do not celebrate the 1940's as a halcyon past in medicine. The system exacted sacrifices from the janitors, floor cleaners, cooks, clerks, technicians, aides, nurses and others who labored to keep the hospital going but who were not unionized. As house officers, we may have prided ourselves on providing excellent technical care, but we didn't see anything wrong with long waits for dispensary patients, limited ward visiting hours (to maximize staff convenience), and inpatient stays prolonged so that we could learn from the course of illness or by pursuing "an interesting finding." I confess with shame I did not challenge the view with which we were indoctrinated that free care patients owed us the obligation to make themselves available for "teaching purposes."

As medical capabilities multiplied and as insurance coverage grew, health care costs rose rapidly — from 4.1% of the GNP in 1940 to 4.5% in 1950 and to 6% by the mid-1960's. More to the point, reimbursement for hospitals was on a cost-plus basis. The longer the stay, the more numerous the tests and the consultations, the greater the reimbursement. Costs for new hospital buildings and expensive equipment were amortized against per diem charges. Another jump in revenue came with the passage of Medicare and Medicaid in 1965 during the Johnson Administration. The legislation provided major and much needed benefits to elderly and poor Americans. The bills were savagely opposed by the leaders of organized medicine and by some academics.[10] Nonetheless, the legislation proved to be a bonanza for the profession when the White House, in response to the perceived political power of the AMA, invited its leaders to help fashion reimbursement regulations. The specification of "usual and customary fees" and the perpetuation of a cottage-industry approach turned "losers" into "winners" for doctors and hospitals; free care, for the poor and the elderly, became paid care. I regret to note that all of us — practitioners, academics, administrators and hospital trustees — fed the exponential increase in costs.

We created a pool of funds that attracted corporate entrepreneurs obeying Sutton's Law (Willie Sutton, a career bank robber, was caught and jailed repeatedly. Asked why he continued to rob banks, Willie answered without hesitation: "Because that's where the money is."). The gold rush was on. It led to what economist Eli Ginzberg (1984) termed "the monetarization of medicine;" that is, the penetration of the money economy into all facets of the health care system because of:

> "the opportunities created by <u>faulty public policy</u>, primarily

through reimbursement for those with money-making proclivities to establish a strong niche in what was formerly a quasi-eleemosynary sector…To secure a long-term financial foundation (for innovation, quality, access and equity at an affordable cost), American medicine will require a combination of political leadership and professional cooperation that is not yet visible on the horizon."

For-profit managed care organizations (MCOs) recognized a prime opportunity to make a killing and moved aggressively into the marketplace. In 1985, 75% of HMO members were in not-for-profit plans; by 1999, the proportion had fallen to one-third (Himmelstein *et al.* 2001). Some pioneering non-profit HMOs (like HIP and HCHP) either had to sell out or change from a staff model to payments per service provided. High quality HMOs (like Kaiser-Permanente) began to experience unsustainable losses and had to reduce staffing patterns. Between 1970 and 1998, the number of health administrators increased more than 24 fold while the number of MDs, RN, and other clinical personnel increased only 2.5 fold. If the U.S. reduced its administrative workforce in health to Canada's level (on a per capita basis) we would employ 1.4 million fewer managers and clerks (Himmelstein *et al.* 2001). MCO CEOs rake in huge compensation packages; the 10 highest paid executives in the managed care industry received an average of $1.7 million dollars each in the year 2000!

Fifteen years ago, as MCOs began to dominate the medical marketplace, John McKinlay and John Arches (1985) wrote a prophetic paper about the "proletarianization" of the American physician. As physicians lost control of the "means of production" to corporate managers of the health system, they became wage laborers subject to the control and incentives of the owners of the commodified health system. With growth in size, organizational centralization becomes more prominent; decision making is further and further removed from the sites where physicians care for patients. To the extent physicians become executives in the new systems and rise in the hierarchy, they behave less and less like physicians and more like managers.

Managed care touts itself as the solution for rising Medicare costs. Is it? What it succeeds at is cream-skimming. Managed care organizations make their bundle by enrolling *healthy* Medicare eligibles; ill recipients disenroll once sickness ensues because choice of physician and availability of care are both sharply restricted. Health Care Financing Administration data reveal that disenrollment varies with the profit status of the plans. Nine of the 10 plans with the lowest rates were not-for-profit; 7 of the 10 with the highest rates of disenrollment were for-profit (Families USA Foundation 1997). As taxpayer costs for the disenrolled and unenrolled elderly sick rise, managed care has been profiting hugely from retaining healthy seniors (Morgan *et al.* 1997).

There is simply no way at all that an academic health science center can maintain excellence in clinical care, serve impecunious patients, teach students and residents, advance the science of medicine, and compete for price with for-profit hospitals that do not teach or do research and are willing to provide care no better than they need to, as long as they can do so at a profit (Iezzoni 1997). Graduate medical education is centered in fewer than 1500 of the nation's 7000 hospitals; 100 of them provide almost half of residency training (Commonwealth Fund 1985). Clinical research in teaching hospitals entails costs beyond those defrayed by grants. Analysis of extramural grant awards reveals an inverse relationship between penetration of the "medical market" by MCOs and the likelihood that medical schools situated within those "market areas" compete successfully for National Institutes of Health Awards (Moy *et al.* 1997). Potential investigators in such schools have less "protected time" because they are obliged to carry greater patient care responsibilities (Campbell *et al.* 1997). Costs at academic medical centers are approximately 44% higher than those for non-teaching hospitals because of teaching intensity (Mechanic *et al.* 1998). Without substantial subsidies from an all-payer fund, academic medical centers are nonstarters in a competitive medical marketplace.

Some MCOs have engaged in clearly illegal if not criminal behavior. Columbia/HCA, the largest for-profit hospital chain, had to sack its CEO in response to a federal criminal investigation of its practices (Eichenwald 1997a; Sharpe 1997). That included maintaining two sets of books, one for its own accounting purposes and a second to justify overcharges to the government. It pressured its physicians to invest in its hospitals so they would have a financial stake in referrals; it provided cash bonuses to its executives if they met financial targets (Eichenwald 1997; Rodriguez 1998).

Can managed care be credited with moderating recent year-to-year increases in medical care costs? Only in small part. The principal engines of cost containment were (1) the power of large employers to force lower premiums, (2) collective purchasing of health insurance by business coalitions at sizable discount, (3) surplus bed capacity in hospitals, (4) a weak physicians' labor market that left "sellers" at the mercy of proxy "buyers" in the medical market place, and (5) competition between delivery organizations (Ginzberg and Ostow 1997).

Increasing health care expenditures are inexorable because of the aging of the population, a labor intensive health sector, and most important of all, technological innovation and the resulting greater capabilities of medicine (Newhouse 1992). Examples of highly desirable and very costly developments (none of them available when I was an intern) are heart surgery, renal dialysis, joint replacement, organ transplantation, new imaging methods (CTs, MRIs, PETs, MEGs) and more effective but more expensive drugs. About 10% of the 200 biggest selling prescription drugs are new each year (Weissbrod 1991). Despite government price negotiations, Canada's prescription drug bill has soared nearly 350% during the past 15 years (Kondro 2001). Despite a rapid decrease in the average length of hospital stay (LOS) for a given illness, hospital costs for the care of that illness episode have increased. The cost of each day has gone up faster than the LOS has shrunk! The early days of hospitalization cost the most because of high-tech interventions. It is the relatively inexpensive "convalescent" days that are being eliminated. As LOS goes down, stress on house officers goes up; new admissions demand much more physician input than recovery days (Dellit *et al.* 2001).

## Psychiatric Coverage

Why did insurance coverage for in-patient medical treatment exclude psychiatric care? Private insurance was an innovation in the U.S. initiated by a Texas teachers' union in 1929. At that time, serious mental illness meant custodial hospitalization in state and county mental institutions. Insurance plans guaranteed subscribers access to participating member hospitals; that is, general hospitals. For the most part, those hospitals did not have psychiatric beds; hence, there was no coverage.

In the 1950's and '60's, when psychiatric in-patient stays became brief because of the availability of psychotropic drugs, many general hospitals (which had unfilled general medical beds) opened psychiatric units. Blue Cross and other insurance plans extended coverage for admission to those units, commonly for up to 30 days (Reed *et al.* 1972). Psychiatric hospitals also became eligible for reimbursement and the number of private treatment beds rose steadily from 14,300 in 1970 to 43,700 in 1992 (before falling to 33,600 in 1998) (Center for Mental Health Services 1998). Chains of private psychiatric hospitals proliferated as separate entities were purchased. By the mid-'80s their profits had become so enormous that they were touted as an investment opportunity by a leading brokerage firm. One "advantage" of psychiatric hospitals for investors was that the DRGs were never able to be applied because of the much greater variability in the duration of stay for an episode of mental versus medical illness. The psychiatric hospital stay was dependent not only on the nature of the patient's disorder but also on the availability of alternate living arrangements and appropriate treatment in the community.[11]

In the late '80s and '90s, MCOs and indemnity insurers began to limit sharply the length of the hospital stay they would reimburse; the 30 day limit we had protested a decade earlier became a remembrance of things past. Leading psychiatric hospitals teetered on the balance of bankruptcy. Length of stay (LOS) data from two excellent, academically affiliated psychiatric hospitals emphasize the point. In 1986 in hospital A, the average LOS was about 73 days; the number of admissions per year about 1000, and the number of beds 320. By 1992, although average LOS had been cut to 30 days, the institution was still heavily in the red because of unreimbursed days. By 2000, hospital bed capacity had been reduced by half and LOS to 8 days; admissions had increased six fold (yes, to 6000!). The hospital balance sheet remains at the margins (because third-party payors reimburse at less than full cost) but the major hemorrhage from endowment has been staunched. Data from Hospital B are similar: average LOS 45 days in 1990, 24 days in 1992, 14 days in 2000. Some patients who need hospitalization are denied it altogether; others are pushed out prematurely because the insurer will not agree to additional days the staff considers necessary. The rules are designed to improve the bottom line rather than to provide optimum care.

Thus, psychiatry is in the paradoxical position of having much more effective treatments to offer and of being much less able to provide them. The tasks ahead are both organizational and political. The APA tends to conflate the public interest with its professional interest, to function as a guild rather than as an advocate for the public. The challenge is to ally ourselves with other professionals in defense of the health of the public rather than engaging in internecine warfare with psychologists and social workers over hegemony and fees. The epidemiologic evidence is that the need is great. If we focus on meeting that need, psychiatry will have an honorable place in medicine.

Not quite 30 years ago (Eisenberg 1973), I concluded a paper with a bold assertion I now repeat:

> "Psychiatry at its best is a paradigm for the general medical practice of the future. This may seem an outlandish claim for a field which boasts few spectacular advances. Yet I believe it to be true because psychiatric practice deals with human distress in a context that must include the psychosocial as well as the biological. There are no imperialistic aims behind this claim. Quite to the contrary, in so far as psychiatry is successful in clarifying the psychobiological bases of health and illness, that knowledge will pass into the domain of the generalist and the psychiatrist will join other specialists in the secondary and tertiary cadres of the health system."

## REFERENCES


Adam, D. (2001) Flickering light raises possibility of changing "constant." *Nature* 412:757.

American Psychiatric Association (1952) Diagnostic and Statistical Manual of Mental Diseases. First Edition. Washington: American Psychiatric Association Mental Hospital Service.

American Psychiatric Association (1968) Diagnostic and Statistical Manual of Mental Disorders. Second Edition. Washington: American Psychiatric Association.

American Psychiatric Association (1980) Diagnostic and Statistical Manual of Mental Disorders. Third Edition. Washington: American Psychiatric Association.

American Psychiatric Association (1994) Diagnostic and Statistical Manual of Mental Disorders. Fourth Edition. Washington: American Psychiatric Association.

Appel, K.E., Pearson, M. (1959) Facilities for psychiatric education: survey of psychiatric departments in medical schools. *American Journal of Psychiatry* 115:698-705.

Barker, P. (1991) Regeneration. London: Viking; New York: Viking Penguin.

Barzansky, B., Etzel, S.I. (2001) Educational Programs in U.S. Medical Schools 2000-2001. Appendix II Graduate Medical Education. *Journal of the American Medical Association* 286:1095-1107.

Cade, J.F.J. (1949) Lithium salts in the treatment of psychotic excitement. *Medical Journal of Australia* 2:349-52.

Campbell, E.G., Weissman, J.S., Blumenthal, D. (1997) Relationship between market competition and the activities and attitudes of medical school faculty. *Journal of the American Medical Association* 278:222-226.

Canada (1983) Preserving Universal Medicare. Ottawa: Government of Canada

Center for Mental Health Services. Mental Health, United States, 1998. Manderscheid, R.W., Henderson, M.J. (Eds) DHHS Pub. No. (SMA) 99-3285. Washington, DC: Supt. of Docs., U.S. Govt. Print. Off., 1998.

Clark, T. (2001) Taming Africa's Killer Lake. *Nature* 409:554-5.

Cohen, J.D. (2001) ABC's of secondary prevention in CHD: easier said than done. *Lancet* 357: 972-3.

Commonwealth Fund (1985) Prescription for Change: Report of the Task Force on Academic Medical Centers. New York: Commonwealth Fund.

Dellitt, H., Armas-Loughran, B., Busl, G.H., Sepkowitz, K.A., Thaler, H. (2001) A method for assessing house staff workload as a function of length of stay. *Journal of the American Medical Association* 286:1023.

Doll, R. (1991) Development of controlled trials in preventive and therapeutic medicine. *J Biosoc Sci* 23:365-78.

Eichenwald, K. (1997a) Hospital giant, under attack, sets shake up. *New York Times.* August 7: A-1.

Eichenwald, K. (1997b) Hospital chain cheated U.S. on expenses, documents show. *New York Times.* December 18:A-1.

Eisenberg, L. (1962) If not now, when? *American Journal of Orthopsychiatry* 32:781-93.

Eisenberg, L. (1973) The future of psychiatry. *The Lancet* ii:1371-5.

Eisenberg, L. (1986) Mindlessness and brainlessness in psychiatry. *Brit J Psychiat.* 1986; 148:497-508.

Eisenberg, L. (1986) Healthcare: for patients or for profits? *American Journal of Psychiatry* 143;1015-19.

Eisenberg, L. (1992) Treating depression and anxiety in primary care: closing the gap between knowledge and practice. *New England Journal of Medicine*: 326: 1080-4.

Eisenberg, L. (1995) Medicine – molecular, monetary or more than both? *Journal of the American Medical Association* 274: 331-4.

Eisenberg, L. (1998) Nature, niche and nurture: the role of social experience in transforming genotype into phenotype. *Academic Psychiatry*. 1998; 22: 213-222.

Eisenberg, L. (2000) Is psychiatry more mindful or brainier than it was a decade ago? *Brit J Psychiat*. 176-1-5.

Euroaspire II (2001) Life-style and risk-factor management and use of drug therapies in coronary patients from 15 European countries. *European Heart Journal* 22: 554-72.

Families USA Foundation (1997) *Comparing Medical HMOs: Do They Keep Their Members?* Washington, DC: Families USA Foundation.

Frank, J.D. (1961) Persuasion and Healing. Baltimore: The Johns Hopkins Press.

Ginzberg, E. (1984) Monetarization of medical care. *New England Journal of Medicine* 310: 1162-5.

Ginzberg, E., Ostow, M. (1997) Managed care – a look back and a look ahead. *New England Journal of Medicine* 336: 1018-20.

Goldberg, D., Huxley, P. (1992) Common Mental Disorders: A Biosocial Model. London: Routledge.

Grob, G.N. (1994) The Mad Among Us. Cambridge: Harvard University Press.

Grob, G.N. (1983) Mental Illness and American Society 1875-1940. Princeton: Princeton University Press.

Himmelstein, D., Woolhandler, S., Hellander, I. (2001) Bleeding the Patient: The Consequences of Corporate Health Care. Philadelphia, PA: Common Courage Press.

Hogenesch, J.B., Ching, K.A., Batalov, S., *et al.* (2001) A comparison of the Celera and Ensembl predicted gene sets reveals little overlap in novel genes. Cell 106: 413-15.

Iezzoni, L.I. (1997) Major teaching hospitals defying Darwin [editorial]. *Journal of the American Medical Association* 278: 520.

Jahoda, M. The Migration of Psychoanalysis: Its impact on American psychiatry. In Fleming D, Bailyn B (1969) The Intellectual Migration: Europe and American 1930-1960. Cambridge: Belknap Press of Harvard University Press.

Jarvis, E. (1855/1971) Insanity and Idiocy in Massachusetts: Report of the Commission on Lunacy, 1855. 1971 edition with a critical introduction by GN Grob. Cambridge: A Commonwealth Fund Book; Harvard University Press.

Jones, F.D. (2000) Military psychiatry since World War II. In R.W., Menninger, and J.C. Nemiah (Eds) American Psychiatry After World War II. Washington, DC: American Psychiatric Press, Inc.; 3-36.

Jones, M. (1952) The Therapeutic Community. New York: Basic Books.

Kallmann, F. (1946) The genetic theory of schizophrenia: an analysis of 691 schizophrenic twin index families. *Am J Psychiatry* 103: 309-22.

Kast, B. (2001) The best supporting actors. *Nature* 412: 674-678.

Klerman, G.L. (1990) The contemporary American scene: diagnosis and classification of mental disorders. In Sources and Traditions of Classification in Psychiatry (ed. Sartorius, N., Jablensky, A., Regier, D.A., Burke. J.D., Hirschfeld, R.M.A.). Bern: Huber. pp. 93-137.

Kondro, W. (2001) Canadian drive to curb drug expenditures. *Lancet* 358:648.

Kowalczyk, L. (2001) HMO rates climb again for 2002. *Boston Globe* 21 June: A:1.

Kramer, M. (1969) Cross-national study of diagnosis of the mental disorders. *Am J Psych* 125: Suppl I & II.

Kringlen, E. (2000) Twin studies in schizophrenia with special emphasis on concordance figures. *Am J Med Genet* 97:4-11.

Kuhn, R. (1958) The treatment of depressive states with G22355 (Imipramine hydrochloride). *American Journal of Psychiatry* 115:459-64.

Lindley, D. (2001) Book Review. *Nature,* 410:146.

Luhrmann, T. (2000) Of Two Minds. New York: Knopf.

Mechanic, R., Coleman, K., Dobson, A. (1998) Teaching hospital costs: implications for academic missions in a competitive market. *Journal of the American Medical Association* 280: 1015-19.

McKinlay, J.B., Arches, J. (1985) Towards the proletarianization of physicians. *International Journal of Health Services* 15: 161-195.

Meehl, P.E. (1965) Response to Eysenck. *International Journal of Psychiatry* 1: 156-7.

Mitchell, S.W. (1894) Address before the 50th annual meeting of the American Medico-Psychological Association. *Journal of Nervous and Mental Disorders* 21: 413-438.

Morgan, R.O., Virnig, B.A., DeVito, C.A., Persily, N.A. (1997) The Medicare-HMO revolving door – the healthy go in and the sick go out. *New England Journal of Medicine* 337: 169-175.

Moy, E., Mazzaschi, A.J., Levin, R.J., Blake, D.A., Griner, P.F. (1997) Relationship between National Institutes of Health research awards to US medical schools and managed care market penetration. *Journal of the American Medical Association* 278: 217-221.

Newhouse, J.P. (1992) Medical care costs: how much welfare loss? *Journal of Economic Perspectives* 6: 3-21.

Newhouse, J.P. (1993) An iconoclastic view of health cost containment. *Health Affairs Supplement* 153-171.

Odegaard, O. (1964) Patterns of discharge from Norwegian psychiatric hospitals before and after the introduction of psychotropic drugs. *American Journal of Psychiatry* 120: 772-8.

Pasamanick, B. (Ed) (1959). Epidemiology of Mental Disorder. Washington, DC: American Association for the Advancement of Science.

Pearson, K., Moul, M. (1925-26) The problem of alien immigration into Great Britain illustrated by an examination of Russian and Polish Jewish children. *Ann Eugenics* 1:5-127.

Pellmar, T.C. and Eisenberg, L. (Editors) Bridging Disciplines in the Brain, Behavioral and Clinical Sciences. Washington, DC: National Academy Press 2000.

Pressman, J.D. (1998) Last Resort: Psychosurgery and the Limits of Medicine. NY: Cambridge University Press.

Proctor, R. (1988) Racial hygiene: Medicine under the Nazis. Cambridge, MA Harvard University Press pp. 955, 212, 345.

Reed, L.S., Myers, E.S., Schneidemandel, P.L. (1972) Health Insurance and Psychiatric Care: Utilization and Cost. Washington, DC: The American Psychiatric Association.

Regier DA, Goldberg ID, Taube CA (1978) The de facto U.S. mental health services system. *Archives of General Psychiatry* 35: 685-93.

Robins. L.N. (1993) Vietnam veterans' rapid recovery from heroin addiction: a fluke or normal expectation? *Addiction* 88: 1041-1054.

Robins, L.N., Regier, D.A., Editors (1991) Psychiatric Disorders in America: The Epidemiologic Catchment Area Study. New York: The Free Press.

Rodriguez, E.M. (1998) FBI affidavit detail fraud allegations at Columbia/HCA's home health unit. *Wall Street Journal.* February 11: A-3.

Rogow, A. (1970) The Psychiatrists. New York: Putnam.

Scientific Group on Mental Health Research (1964) *Report to the Director General, 6-10 April.* MHO/PA/75.64. Geneva: World Health Organization.

Seife, C. (2001) Changing constants cause controversy. *Science* 293: 1410-11.

Sharfstein, S.S., Muszynski, S., Myers, E. (1984) Health Insurance and Psychiatric Care: Update and Appraisal. Washington, DC: American Psychiatric Press, Inc.

Sharpe, A. (1977) Columbia/HCA confirms departure of another two executives, more expected. *Wall Street Journal.* August 15: B-5.

Shepherd, M., Goodman, N., Watt, D.C. (1961) The application of hospital statistics in the evaluation of pharmacotherapy in a psychiatric population. *Comprehensive Psychiatry* 2: 11-19.

Smith, M.L., Glass, G.V., Miller, T,I. (1980) The Benefits of Psychotherapy. Baltimore: The Johns Hopkins Press.

Srole, L., Langner, T.S., Michael, S.T., Opler, M.K., Rennie, T.A.C. (1962) Mental Health in the Metropolis (Vol. 1) New York: McGraw Hill Book Co.

Stromgren, E. (1994) Recent history of European psychiatry – ideas, developments and personalities: the Annual Eliot Slater Lecture, *Am J Hum Genet* 54:405-410.

Torrey, E.F. (1997) Out of the Shadows: Confronting America's Mental Illness Crisis. New York: Wiley.

Weisbrod, B.A. (1991) The health care quadrilemma: an essay on technological change, insurance, quality of care, and cost containment. *Journal of Economic Literature* 29: 523-552.

Weissman, M.M., (2001) The paradox of psychotherapy: too many, too few; too much, too little In Weissman, M.M. (Editor): Treatment of Depression: Bridging the 21st Century. Washington: American Psychiatric Press. pp. 301-329.

Young, A. (1995) The Harmony of Illusions: Inventing Post Traumatic Stress Disorder. Princeton: Princeton University Press.

## Footnotes

1. They were so classified in the first edition of the Diagnostic and Statistical Manual (1952): "Disorders of psychogenic origin or without clearly defined tangible cause or structural change." DSM II (1968) distinguished between psychoses associated with organic brain syndromes and those that were "not attributed to physical conditions." As late as DSM IIIR (1987), the official manual included the category: Organic Mental Disorders as a major axis separate from schizophrenia and mood disorders. Not until DSM IV (1994) was the term organic mental disorder specifically disavowed "because it implies that 'non-organic' mental disorders do not have a biological basis" (p. 123).

2. The enthusiasm for psychiatry was eroded by a new commitment to primary care in the era of social activism resulting from Vietnam. "People-oriented" medical students who were weighing careers in psychiatry (I chatted with many in the '60s and '70s) opted for primary care on the expectation they could intervene medically and psychologically. My warnings that the economics of primary care (the press of cost controls was already evident) would leave them precious little time to take a thorough history, let alone provide counseling, were unavailing.

3. The new diagnostic scheme is a major advance over DSM-I and II. But with each iteration it becomes more fragmented and bureaucratized. It has become an industry – and a profitable one at that for the A.P.A. which makes tens of millions of dollars with each new edition – because a DSM-IV code is the precondition for reimbursement. The situation has begun to resemble the debate among three umpires about the meaning of balls and strikes in the great American game of baseball. The first, a modest man, claimed only: "I calls 'em as I sees 'em." The second, an arrogant and officious man, insisted: "I calls 'em as they is!" The third, a man of philosophic bent, dismissed their comments with: "They may be balls, they may be strikes, but they ain't nothin' until I call 'em!"

4. The Society for Neuroscience, founded in 1969, had 1000 members in 1970. It was interdisciplinary in that its founders were neuroanatomists, neurochemists, neurophysiologists, neuropharmacologists, brain imagers and clinical scientists: neurologists and psychiatrists. In the past 30 years, membership has multiplied 25 fold! Meetings have become a challenge to organize, getting from one session to another an exercise in agility and the camaraderie of earlier years is efflorescing. The growth of the Society has been so prodigious, the territory it covers so broad, and the methods it employs so varied that neuroscience itself is beginning to fragment into subdisciplines, of which cognitive neuroscience is an instance.

5. Maternal care is literally embodied in the development of the child by two-way traffic between genes and behavior. In rodents, maternal licking, grooming, and nursing behavior (LGN) is a major determinant of endocrine and behavioral responses. Adult offspring of high LGN mothers are less fearful and show diminished hypothalamic-pituitary-adrenal responses to stress. Female offspring of high LGN dams themselves exhibit high LGN maternal behavior when they become dams. One might suppose transmission is genetic. However, when female pups born to low LGN dams are cross-fostered to high LGN dams, they become high LGN with their own pups. Maternal behavior has been transmitted across generations by "culture" but that culture has regulated gene expression in brain regions controlling stress responses (Francis *et al.* 1999). Equally illuminating is the contrasting example provided by the vole (Young *et al.* 1999). Vole species vary markedly in their social behavior. The prairie vole is social and monogamous, the montane vole asocial and promiscuous. In the male prairie vole mating stimulates a secretion of the hormone arginine vasopressin (AVP). The release of AVP is associated with pair-bonding and maternal care; blockade of its receptor in the brain prevents both bonding and parenting responses to mating. In contrast, administration of AVP has no such effect on the montane vole. The molecular explanation is clear; the montane vole reception gene lacks a 428 base-pair coding sequence found in the prairie vole gene. Here, gene structures determine and refract behavior patterns.

6. This now seems obvious, but it wasn't evident to those of us who served on the Scientific Group on Mental Health Research charged with drawing up a research agenda for the W.H.O. Office of Mental Health in 1964. Our 10 recommendations were suitable enough but not one was directed at mental health services in primary care! True, that meeting was held 14 years before the W.H.O. Alma Ata Declaration on Health for All. As a participant, I continue to be astonished that primary care was so far below the horizon of our vision that none of the participants nor either of our distinguished Co-chairs (Robert Felix, Director of the NIMH, and Sir Aubrey Lewis, Director of the Maudsley Hospital), recognized the key role of the primary care system to effective mental health services (Scientific Group 1964).

7. In Pat Barker's splendid novel (Regeneration) she imaginatively reconstructs an actual encounter between the psychiatrist W.H.R. Rivers (a founder of British anthropology) and the soldier-poet Siegfried Sassoon at the casualty hospital, Craiglockhart. Rivers' articles on the psychogenic origins of war neuroses were widely read and he established a course in psychological medicine for doctors in the military. Barker indicts the political use of psychiatric terminology (long before its application in the USSR). Sassoon, an officer decorated for his bravery in combat, violated the command structure by sending a letter to the London Times calling the slaughter of men in trench warfare in France senseless. Because ordering a court martial for a bemedalled hero would have given further publicity to his critique, Sassoon was designated "a psychiatric case" and sent back to the casualty hospital. Barker skillfully highlights Rivers' moral distress as a psychiatrist charged with restoring his patients to mental health in order to send them back to slaughter.

8. The United States is unique in that clinically trained psychologists, social workers, and other mental health clinicians far outnumber psychiatrists. According to data from the NIMH Survey and Analysis Branch (2001), there are only some 41,000 clinically trained psychiatrists in the U.S. in contrast to about 77,000 clinical psychologists, 96,000 social workers, and 83,000 registered nurses in mental health organizations. In addition, there are 108,000 counselors and 44,000 marriage and family therapists. Because psychologists and social workers are eligible for reimbursement as independent providers of care and because counselors are employed to provide care by managed care organizations, competition in the U.S. mental health "market place" is intense. The professional societies representing each group joust over hegemony.

   For comparison, England (excluding Scotland, Wales, and Northern Ireland) with a population of 50 million has about 6400 psychiatrists (2600 of them consultants), 4700 psychologists, (including trainees) and 36,000 qualified psychiatric nurses, whom Professor David Goldberg regards as "the mainstay of U.K. mental health services" (personal communication 2001).

9. These salaries must be seen in relation to medical school tuition; it was $400 when I was a student at Penn in the 40's and it will be $29,000 at Harvard for 2001-02; estimated cost of attendance budget figures for years one to four (educational costs plus living expenses) are $46,500 for the first, $51,000 for the second, $49,250 for the third and $46,850 for the fourth year. Thus, the cost of a medical education at Harvard Medical School comes to about $194,000 (the lowest of the three private schools in Boston!). Tuition at University of Massachusetts Medical School (a state school) is $8,352; total cost (tuition plus living expenses) for a medical education at UMass is calculated at $120,000. About 60% of all American medical students attend state schools. Nonetheless, medical graduates carry an average debt load at graduation of $85,000, a major impediment to an academic career. With interest forbearance during residency training, repayment costs can be as high as $900 a month on a 20-year plan or $775 on a 30-year plan.

10. During the political campaign for insurance coverage for the poor and the elderly, Robert Cooke, Helen Taussig and I in the Department of Pediatrics at Hopkins signed our names to an advertisement for Medicaid and Medicare in the Baltimore Sun. For weeks afterward, the doctors' dining room (we still had one in '65!) was an uncomfortable place to be because some "colleagues" would not acknowledge my presence by deigning to greet me. That, however, was hardly a surprise and no more

than a minor nuisance. Much more bothersome was a claque of faculty and medical students who believed we had signed the ad in order to get more federal grants! Motivated as they were by their own self-interest, they projected their world view onto others.

11. In an October 1984 advisory to its clients entitled: "The Psychiatry Hospital Industry," Salomon Brothers, a Wall Street brokerage firm, reported to its clients that:

> "The psychiatric hospital industry is an attractive sub-segment... for investors. In-patient psychiatric care is widely insured, occurs with predictable and increasing incidence and is complex enough to r*ender cost-control efforts difficult*...[additional] advantages over general hospitals include the widespread acceptance of *two classes of psychiatric care: high quality care in private psychiatric hospitals...versus lower quality care in government-owned mental health centers*." (Italics added).

What enchanted stock brokers was the difficulty in implementing cost-control because of imprecision in diagnosis, "the major role of environmental factors," "lack of standardized treatment," and "inability to measure the extent of recovery." What was bad for patients was good for investors.

# Relevance of Epidemiology for Intervention in Mental Disorders

**Kathleen R. Merikangas, Ph.D.**
**Mood and Anxiety Disorders Program, National Institute of Mental Health, Intramural Research Program —**

**Beatrix Hamburg, M.D.**
**Cornell Medical College**

## I. Introduction

By the year 2020, it is estimated that psychiatric and neurologic disorders will account for 15% of the total burden of all diseases. Major depression is the leading cause of disability among those age five and over, and the second leading source of disease burden surpassing cardiovascular diseases, dementia, lung cancer and diabetes (Murray & Lopez, 1996). The dramatic impact of mood disorders, schizophrenia, and substance abuse and anxiety disorders on lifetime disability highlights the importance of epidemiology in surveillance, understanding and control of the major mental disorders. The goals of this paper are to: (1) *describe the goals and tools of epidemiology*, (2) *discuss the application of the epidemiologic method to mental disorders*; (3) *present the magnitude of mental disorders in the population*; (4) *review the major risk factors for mental disorders*; (5) *present a summary of the role of epidemiology in identifying the role of genetic risk factors*; and (6) *discuss the implications of epidemiology for prevention of mental disorders and substance use disorders.*

## II. Overview of the Discipline of Epidemiology

*Definition and Study Designs*. Epidemiology is defined as the study of the distribution and determinants of diseases in human populations. Epidemiologic studies are concerned with the extent and types of illnesses in groups of people and with the factors that influence their distribution (Mausner and Balm, 1984). Researchers in this domain are concerned with the role of both intrinsic and extrinsic factors, consisting of interactions that may occur between the host, agent, and environment, the classic triangle of epidemiology, to produce a disease state. This is an excellent model for conceptualizing drug abuse which has a clear agent, but less relevant for depression, anxiety, schizophrenia and behavior disorders which lack clear evidence for the role of environmental agents in their etiology. The ultimate goal of epidemiologic studies is to identify the etiology of a disease and thereby prevent or intervene in its progression.

In order to achieve this goal, epidemiologic studies generally proceed from descriptive studies which specify the amount and distribution of a disease within a population by person, place, and time (that is, descriptive epidemiology), to more focused studies of the determinants of disease in specific groups (that is, analytic epidemiology) (Mausner and Balm, 1984).

Descriptive epidemiologic studies are important in specifying the rates and distribution of disorders in the general population. These data can be applied to identify biases that may exist in treated populations and to construct case registries from which persons may serve as probands for analytic epidemiologic studies. Such attention to sampling issues is a major contribution of the epidemiologic approach, as individuals identified in clinical settings often constitute the tip of the iceberg of the disease and may not be representative of the general population of similarly affected individuals with respect to demographic, social, or clinical characteristics. Associations which are identified at the descriptive level are then tested systematically with case-control designs that compare the relationship between a particular disease risk factor and correlate with the presence or absence of a given disease, after controlling for relevant confounding variables. Case-control studies usually involve a retrospective design to investigate these particular associations, and then proceed to prospective cohort studies which can actually test the direction of such associations.

The identification of risk factors for a disease comprise an intermediate step in the process of identifying a discrete and valid disorder in the general population, and culminate in the conducting of analytic studies that attempt to identify etiologic factors. There are several criteria for assessing the extent to which a risk factor is causally involved in a trait or disease. These include the strength of the association, a dose-response effect, and a lack of temporal ambiguity. Broader criteria that can be applied to a set of studies on a putative etiologic risk factor include: consistency of the findings; biologic plausibility of the hypothesis; and the specificity of association (Kleinbaum *et al.*, 1982). Each of these analytic approaches is germane to epidemiologic research and can be applied to the field of psychiatry to identify risk factors for mental disorders and potential mechanisms of etiology.

## III. Application of Epidemiology to Psychiatry

Descriptive community studies have been conducted throughout the world over the past 100 years. The rich clinical description in some of the classic studies, particularly in Scandinavia, has been unparalleled in recent research. **Table 1** presents a more complete description of the major goals of epidemiologic investigations in psychiatry.

**TABLE 1.**

**Goals of Epidemiologic Studies**

- Develop Standardized Assessments of Psychiatric Disorders
- Establish Validity of Diagnostic Nomenclature
- Establish Magnitude of Psychiatric Disorders in the General Population
- Identify Risk and Protective Factors for Psychopathology
- Collect Information on Patterns of Use and Adaquacy of Psychiatric Services
- Provide Empirical Basis for Timing and Targets for Prevention

***Definitions and Assessment of Psychiatric Disorders*.** One of the major contributions of psychiatric epidemiology during the past few decades has been the establishment of reliable methods for defining and assessing psychiatric disorders including standardized structured and semi-structured diagnostic interviews (Robins, 1992; Henderson, 1996). There now are numerous structured interviewers designed for use by lay interviewers that may serve as screeners for contemporary diagnostic criteria including the Diagnostic Interview Survey (Robins *et al.*, 1981), its successor, the Composite International Diagnostic Interview (Robins *et al.*, 1988) which acquires information for both the DSM and ICD criteria, and the Diagnostic Interview Survey for Children (DISC), for children (Shaffer *et al.*, 19). The most widely-used semi-structured interviews for use by clinically experienced interviewers include the Structured Clinical Interview for DSM-Ill-R (Spitzer *et al.*, 1992), Schedule for Affective Disorder and Schizophrenia (SADS) (Endicott and Spitzer, 1972), several ancillary interviews for use in specialized settings, and the Kiddie-SADS (Orvaschel *et al.*, 1982) for youth. Data collected with these tools in community surveys provide essential information on the reliability and validity of operationalized diagnostic entities in the general population. The refinement of diagnostic nosology through community study data is typically accomplished by a “bootstrapping” process, whereby epidemiologic findings incrementally lead to more reliable and valid classifications of disorder (which, in turn, improve the accuracy of epidemiologic data) (Eaton & Merikangas, 2000).

***Classification of Psychiatric Disorders***. The first set of criteria in psychiatry that recognizably conformed to this operational pattern in the U.S. were developed by Robins and his colleagues at Washington University in 1972, and became widely known as the "Feighner criteria" (Feighner *et al.*, 1972). Parallel development in the United Kingdom yielded the Present State Examination (PSE), a psychiatric interview designed to standardize the ICD criteria for psychiatric disorders (Wing *et al.*, 1974). Other sets of operational criteria rapidly followed from other groups, culminating in publication of the recent World Health Organization's ICD10 (World Health Organization, 1993) and the American Psychiatric Association's DSM-IV (American Psychiatric Association, 1994).

Data from epidemiologic and primary care settings provided an empirical basis for the development of both of these contemporary diagnostic systems.

The results of community studies have also illustrated the need for further development of the psychiatric diagnostic system (Regier *et al.*, 1990; Kessler *et al.*, 1994). The findings of inadequate coverage of current systems in community and primary care settings, the tendency for comorbidity to be more common than single disorders, and the lack of longitudinal stability of the major diagnostic categories have generated new research designed to examine the thresholds and boundaries of the major psychiatric disorders (*e.g.* Angst & Merikangas, 1997; Kessler *et al.*, 1994). In his discussion of the validity of the psychiatric disorders, Kendell (1989) noted that it is unlikely that the etiologic secrets of the major psychiatric disorders will be unlocked without accurate and valid identification of the syndromes themselves. Such validation has particular relevance for the search for biologic markers, which depend in large part on the identification of discrete and homogeneous forms of disorder (Freedman, 1984).

Another contribution of epidemiology is identification of potential biases in clinical samples that may compromise their generalizability. Samples of contemporary clinical trials in psychiatry are becoming increasingly atypical due to both highly exclusive entry criteria, often to maximize the "purity" of the disorders, and nonsystematic ascertainment source. In fact, the increasing trend towards recruitment of patients for clinical trials through the media (with some advertisements even including screening criteria in the advertisement!) is an epidemiologist's nightmare. Community studies may yield information on biases of samples identified in clinical settings, which are often not representative of the general population of similarly affected individuals with respect to demographic, social, or clinical characteristics.

## IV. Magnitude of Psychiatric Disorders in the General Population.

During the past three decades, psychiatric epidemiologic investigations have flourished. Population base rates can differ dramatically according to the diagnostic definitions and methods of assessment. Population prevalence estimates of mental disorders are available from numerous community surveys throughout the world. Median base rates of the major mental disorders across international studies are 1% for schizophrenia; 1% bipolar affective disorder; 10% major depression; 12% anxiety disorder; and 12% substance use disorder.

**Table 2** presents findings from several of the most recent large-scale community surveys of adult mental disorders that have used structured diagnostic interviews. The largest of the studies, the Epidemiologic Catchment Area program (ECA), sampled community and institutionalized residents from numerous cities across the United States (representing a nearly five-fold increase in sample size over previous North American studies; see Freedman, 1984). More recently, the results of the National Comorbidity Survey (NCS) have become available, and the completion of additional large-scale studies has

**TABLE 2.**

**Lifetime prevalence rates of mental disorders in U.S. Community Surveys**

| | Lifetime Prevelance Rates (SE) by Investigation | |
|---|---|---|
| **Disorder** | **ECA (Robins *et al.*, 1984)** | **NCS (Kessler *et al.*, 1994)** |
| Anxiety Disorders | 15.5 (0.7) | 24.9 (0.8) |
| Affective Disorders | 7.9 (0.6) | 19.3 (0.7) |
| Psychosis (Non-Affective) | 1.7 (0.3) | 0.7 (0.1) |
| Substance Use Disorders | 16.7 (0.8) | 26.6 (1.0) |
| Any Disorders | 32.6 (1.0) | 48.0 (1.1) |

*ECA indicates Epidemiologic Catchment Area;*
*NCS indicates National Comorbidity Survey*

provided important information about the generalizability of assessment methods as well as potential cultural influences on psychopathology rates.

Perhaps the most basic finding from these diverse investigations is the high prevalence of psychiatric disorders in community residents. As demonstrated by the table, the lifetime prevalence rates range from approximately 33% to 48% of the general population. The generally higher NCS rates are likely to be due to the application of increasingly sophisticated interview methods that minimize biases in retrospective recall. Nonetheless, the high prevalence rates across sites underscore the magnitude of psychopathology in non-clinically derived samples. These investigations have added to psychiatry not only by portraying the natural history of these disorders in a descriptive sense, but also by raising important issues about the comparability of clinical and community samples concerning treatment utilization, and the universal nature of psychiatric conditions. Despite the high prevalence rates of mental disorders, it is estimated that 9% of all U.S. adults have mental disorders with significant functional impairment, and 2.6 % have severe and persistent mental disorders (Kessler *et al.*, 1996). However, only a minority of those with major mental disorders receive mental health services, with estimates ranging from 10-20% in a particular year (*Surgeon General Report, 1999*).

The rates shown in Table 2 do not account for the large magnitude of overlap across diagnostic categories that have been consistently demonstrated in community studies. Community studies are a particularly important source of investigation of mechanisms for comorbidity, since those with comorbidity have greater representation in the treatment sector. For example, Angst *et al.*, in press, examined the clinical and research significance of the high frequency of multiple diagnoses emanating from the non-hierarchical descriptive approach to classification in the current diagnostic systems. Data from a 15-year prospective cohort study of young adults from the general community were employed to evaluate the frequency of multiple diagnoses, and the extent to which patterns of multiple diagnoses are associated with indicators of severity of psychopathology. The findings indicated that there was an average number of lifetime disorders in this community-based sample was 2.1 with a range from 0 to 7. Associations within diagnostic spectra were more common than those between diagnostic spectra. The results confirm the link between comorbidity and severity, and further show that there is a direct increase in nearly all of the indicators of severity by the number of disorders for which the subjects met criteria across 15 years. Each of the major diagnostic categories, particularly depression, contributed to increased severity rather than representing a nonspecific effect of the number of disorders.

***Ongoing Research***. NIMH is now supporting a rich series of studies to follow up on the cross-sectional findings of the surveys presented above. Subjects who participated in the ECA are being followed at 10-year intervals (William Eaton, Principal Investigator); likewise, there is currently a 10-year follow up underway of the sample from the original National Comorbidity Survey (Ronald Kessler, Principal Investigator). In addition, new national probability samples with greater ethnic diversity than those of prior samples using measures tailored to the cultural subgroups under investigation are being collected. These studies are collecting data to apply broader diagnostic characterization, to examine more comprehensive measures of risk factors and services (R. Kessler *et al*.; J Jackson *et al*; and M. Allegria *et al*., Principal Investigators). Finally, the first national probability survey of adolescents is now underway as part of the 2000 National Comorbidity Survey Replication (Ronald Kessler, Kathleen Merikangas, and Shelli Avenevoli). A total of 8,700 adolescents drawn from both the general population and school samples are being evaluated.

***International Research***. Although there have been multiple attempts to integrate community studies across the world (Merikangas *et al*., 1996; Merikangas *et al*., 1998; Weissman *et al*., 1996), differences in sampling and methods precluded derivation of true international rates and patterns of disorders. A recent initiative under the joint auspices of the National Institute of Mental Health (Ronald Kessler, Principal Investigator) and World Health Organization (Bedirhan Ustun, Principal Investigator) has been developed to collect parallel data on the base rates of mental disorders in 29 countries in North America, Latin America, Asia, Europe and Africa. Using a common instrument, the W.H.O. CIDI (Robins *et al*., 1987), data will be available on descriptive epidemiology, service use, impact of mental and physical disorders and their interaction, comorbidity, predictors of outcome and the global burden of each of the mental disorders.

***Magnitude of Mental Disorders in Children***. The power of psychiatric epidemiology to enhance our understanding of mental disorders is also evident in its application to childhood mental disorders. Similar to the contributions made in recent years relative to adult psychiatric disorders, there is accumulating community-based data concerning childhood psychopathology. The rate-limiting step in child psychiatry continues to be our lack of classification (and hence, measurement) of childhood disorders, patterns of expression across different developmental stages, and early signs that are predictive of later, lifelong psychopathology. However, the epidemiologic approach can advance knowledge through the collection of information on early signs and risk factors gleaned from high-risk studies, as well as studies on protective factors and processes related to the development of psychopathology in childhood (Dulcan, 1996). Indeed, some of the most important advances in child psychiatry have been through careful work of child psychiatric epidemiologists. Beginning in the 1960's with the Isle of Wight study (for a review, see Rutter, 1989), the importance of often subtle nosological definitions in determining rates of childhood disorders became evident, as well as the importance of complex issues such as diagnostic comorbidity and the relationship between age of onset to correlates of psychiatric syndromes. Similar to adult psychiatric epidemiology, however, the major limitation of this groundbreaking research was the lack of modern diagnostic criteria and assessment methods.

***Methodological Issues in Children.*** The major controversy in the assessment of both adults and children concern definitions of the thresholds distinguishing clinically significant from the normative range of expression of particular symptoms. Using 15-year prospective data on a community-based sample beginning in late adolescence, Angst and Merikangas (2000) have recently presented evidence that depression in youth is better reflected as a dimension rather than categorical measures of the components of depressive disorder. Empirical studies have generally applied adult thresholds to children and adolescents, with the exception of a shorter required duration for some syndromes. Evaluation of appropriate thresholds in youth is confounded by normal developmental changes in patterns of expression of emotion, cognition and behavior.

An extensive literature documents strong psychometric properties of dimensional self-report checklists in community surveys of children and adolescents (for reviews, see Orvaschel, 1985 and Roberts *et al.*, 1991). However, there is poor specificity at the top end of these scales, with most of the youngsters with high scores failing to meet diagnostic criteria for particular disorders. Structured and semi-structured diagnostic interviews have also been developed to assess child and adolescent disorders (*e.g.*, Orvaschel *et al.*, 1982; Chambers *et al.*, 1985; Angold *et al.*, 1995; Shaffer *et al.*, 1996). Diagnostic interviews resolve the uncertainty setting cut points in dimensional scales because they employ explicit rules for assessing syndromes in terms of frequency, duration, and impairment. These diagnostic interviews and rules have made it possible to characterize a definitive set of criteria such that all persons meeting these standards will be uniformly defined as comparable cases. However, two important difficulties unique to the application of structure interviews with youth include the need to interview multiple respondents regarding children, usually including a parent, a teacher, and the child or adolescent, and the lack of sufficiently explicit guidelines regarding a number of required classification distinctions, such as "clinically significant," impairment and "marked" distress (Angold *et al.*, 1995).

***Prevalence of Childhood Disorders.*** Because there are no national data on the prevalence of DSM-N mental disorders in children, the results of a small-scale community-based study of youth are presented in **Table 3** (Shaffer *et al.*, 1996). The one-year prevalence of all

**TABLE 3**

**Prevalance Rates of Mental Disorders in Youth**

| Disorder | Rate | Disorder | Rate |
|---|---|---|---|
| Anxiety | 13.0% | Substance Use Disorder | 2.0% |
| Mood | 6.2% | ANY DISORDER | 20.9% |
| Disruptive Behavior | 10.3% | | |

the major classes of mental disorders with impairment was 20.9%, with anxiety disorders being the most common disorder leading to impairment among youth ages 9 to 17. Substance use disorders were relatively rare in this age group, despite the evidence from other surveys of the high rates of substance use. Costello (1989) reviewed several recent community studies of childhood psychopathology using standardized diagnostic criteria and structured diagnostic interviews (Anderson *et al.*, 1987; Bird *et al.*, 1988; Cohen & Brook, 1987; Costello *et al.*, 1988; Boyle *et al.*, 1987; Offord *et al.*, 1987). The lifetime prevalence rate for one or more DSM-III disorders reported by these studies ranged from 17.6% to 22.0% of children, with internalizing disorders (*e.g.* separation anxiety, phobia, depression) showing the highest prevalence rates. Despite the relatively consistent rates across studies for any childhood disorder, considerable variation was nonetheless found for specific diagnoses. For example, the prevalence of attention deficit disorder ranged from 2.2% to 9.9%, and rates of simple phobia ranged from 2.4% to 9.2%. Such discrepancies may be due in part to differences in rules for the aggregation of disorder reports across child and adult informants, or to variances in the ages of children in the samples. However, an important point raised by Costello (1989) is that while data collected in these studies may have been initially analyzed by different decision rules (thus contributing to discrepancies in prevalence rates), the use of modern data collection methods provides detailed information about individual symptoms. This advance should permit researchers to re-examine data from diverse investigations while applying uniform decision rules.

Approximately 5 to 9% of children ages 9 to 17 suffer from severe emotional disturbances (Friedman *et al.*, 1996). The proportion of youth with severe disturbances is very low in early childhood and rises to adult levels in the late teens (*Surgeon General Report, 1999*). These findings suggest that effort for prevention would best be targeted to youth in the early to late teens, depending upon the age--specific incidence of particular disorders and pathways of disorders.

Community studies also provide important data on patterns of service use. Similar to adults, about 5 to 7% of children receive mental health services in a given year. Unfortunately, there is large variation by ethnicity, with those in greatest need being least likely to be in treatment (*Surgeon General Report, 1999*).

## V. Risk Factors and Correlates of Mental Disorders.

At first glance, epidemiologic investigations may appear distant from the immediate goals of biological and laboratory-based studies of psychopathology. However, epidemiologic studies not only provide estimates of base rates of disorders in the general population, but also key indications of demographic correlates of psychiatric conditions that may be used to guide neurobiological investigations. **Table 4** summarizes the major individual and contextual risk factors and correlates of psychiatric disorders that have been identified in controlled retrospective or prospective cohort studies.

**TABLE 4**

**Risk Factors and Correlates of Mental Disorders**

- Sex
- Age
- Social class
- Family History
- Temperament
- Parental or Early Childhood Insult, Trauma
- Exposure to Toxins
- Exposure to Chronic or Acute Stress
- Physical Illness
- Non-Intact family
- Family Disfunction
- Social disadvantage

The most widely studied correlate of mental disorders is the consistent gender difference in the manifestation of emotional and behavioral disorders. Whereas women having greater rates of anxiety, affective and eating disorders, men report more substance disorders and other behavior disorders. While the sex ratio for the major psychoses is approximately equal, research has also revealed gender differences in the age at onset of schizophrenia (Hafner *et al.*, 1993). Furthermore, investigations across the life span reveal that sex differences in the affective and emotional disorders tend to emerge during adolescence, whereas males tend to have increased rates of behavior and attention problems throughout life (Loeber, 1991; Costello, 1989). In addition, studies of the longitudinal evolution of psychopathology have revealed that anxiety states and depression may result from common underlying biologic and cultural factors with age-dependent expression (Merikangas & Angst, 1996).

The windows of risk for most of the major mental disorders have been well established through accumulation of retrospective data from clinical and community samples as well as prospective studies of youth. The insidious onset of most mental disorders precludes careful dating of incidence, particularly for continua underlying the components of disorders such as depression and anxiety, as well as imprecise thresholds between affected and unaffected status (Angst & Merikangas, 1997). However, the results of community studies reveal that the onset of many of the most common mental disorders is far earlier than previously believed.

***Contextual Risk Factors.*** There has been a long tradition of studies of the role of life events and stress in the development of psychiatric disorders (Brown *et al.*, 1978). Prospective studies of the role of life events and acute stressors have demonstrated that individual characteristics such as personality and proximal contextual factors determine the effect of such stressors in inducing mental disorders. There is now an emerging consensus that environmental stressors tend to precipitate and maintain episodes of psychiatric disorders rather than being of etiologic significance (Henderson, 1996).

Advances in several areas have led to far more complex models of risk. Of particular significance is emerging evidence in the neurosciences regarding the role of experience in molding neural pathways and influencing gene expression. For example, the research of Francis *et al.* (1999) demonstrates the role of environmental manipulation in inducing nongenomic behavioral transmission of stress reactivity in rodents.

Recent twin research also illustrates the strong bi-directional influence between genes and environment in the development of psychiatric disorders (Kendler, 1995). However, the bulk of this work has been based on retrospective and ecological data, and prospective confirmation of this association is still lacking. Such prospective longitudinal studies are critical to evaluate the order of onset of putative risk factors and diseases, as well as to characterize the evolution, course and sequelae of psychiatric disorders.

Other biologic risk factors include exposure to exogenous agents, such as viruses, CNS toxins, physical illnesses, and other exposures that occur at any time after conception. Concerning other environmental factors, one of the most important findings in recent epidemiologic research supports the role of prenatal viral exposure and other possible environmental insults in the development of schizophrenia (Bromet *et al.*, 1995). Likewise, the discovery of bacterially influenced disturbances such as obsessive compulsive disorder has generated substantial interest in viral and bacterial risk factors for the mental disorders as well (Garvey *et al.*, 1998).

## VI. Relevance of Epidemiology to Identifying Genetic Risk Factors

> Although experimental species are of great value for the initial identification and functional analysis of complex disease genes, final evidence for the involvement of these genes in human diseases must come from extensive epidemiological studies, preferably in different populations.
>
> — *Peltonen and McKusick (2001)*

One problem with the risk factor-based approach in contemporary epidemiology is the lack of integration of host factors, and particularly genetic vulnerability. Although the goal of epidemiology is to study the interaction between host, agents, and environment, epidemiologists have tended to neglect "host" characteristics other than demographics (Kuller, 1979). However, increasing evidence reveals that environmental risk factors may either potentiate or protect against expression of underlying genetic and biological vulnerability factors. Furthermore, despite their history of independence, the fields of epidemiology and genetics share much common ground. Both are interested in determining the etiology of complex human disorders and predicting familial recurrence risks for such disorders. The advent of the field of genetic epidemiology has served to bridge the gap between the two fields (Morton, 1982).

There are several comprehensive reviews of the evidence from family, twin, and adoption studies regarding the role of genetic factors in the etiology of mental disorders. Ironically, genetic epidemiologic approaches have been applied far more to mental disorders than to any other class of human diseases. **Table 5** presents an updated summary of the average risk ratios derived from studies of each of the mental disorders. The familial recurrence risks are significantly elevated for all of the major mental disorders, irrespective of the sampling and methods employed. The risk ratios are greatest for bipolar disorder and schizophrenia ranging from 6-10, intermediate for substance dependence (average 4-8) and subtypes of anxiety, particularly panic (5%) and lowest for major depression (average of 2-3)

**TABLE 5**

**Risk Factors of Major Mental Disorders Among Relatives in Controlled Family, Twin and Adoption Studies**

| Disorder | Family | Twin | Adoption |
|---|---|---|---|
| Anxiety Disorders | 9.4 | 2.4 | — |
| Bipolar Disorder | 5.5 | 0.6 | 9.2 |
| Major Depression | 6.8 | 2.4 | 1.8 |
| Schizophrenia | 8.9 | 4.4 | 4.3 |
| Substance Use Disorder | 4.5 | 6.3 | 2.1 |

*Family Studies*. Although a review of this literature is beyond the scope of this chapter, there is consistent evidence that nearly all of the mental disorders are familial, and that genetic factors account for a significant proportion of the variance in their etiology. In fact, controlled studies have revealed that a family history is the most potent and consistent risk factor for the development of most of the major psychiatric disorders (Merikangas & Swendsen, 1997).

Even though family study data cannot discriminate between genetic and environmental risk factors, there are several sources of evidence from which one can infer that genes play an important role in familial aggregation. Evaluation of familial recurrence risk as a function of population prevalence (Risch, 1990) can provide insight into underlying genetic models. Whereas X tends to exceed 20 for most autosomal dominant diseases and those for which the genetic basis has been identified, the range of values of X derived from family studies of many complex disorders tend to range from 2 to 5. In general, there is an inverse relationship between the magnitude of the effect of a gene that contributes to disease susceptibility and the population prevalence because of selective disadvantage. Common diseases are far more likely to result from multiple genes or interactions between several predisposing loci (Risch, 1994). In general, the power of linkage and association studies of disorders with X values less than 10 is extremely low.

Decrement in risk according to the degree of genetic relatedness can be examined to detect interactions between several loci. If the risk to second and third degree relatives decreases by more than 50% this implies that more than a single locus must contribute to disease risk, and no single locus can largely predominate. Such interactive effects among loci contributing to the risk for common familial disorders have been demonstrated for cleft lip and palate, diabetes mellitus, multiple sclerosis, and even schizophrenia (Risch, 1994). Other evidence that genetic factors underlie familial aggregation include a dose-response relationship and specificity of familial patterns of disease expression.

***Twin Studies***. Although the traditional application of the twin design focuses on the estimation of the heritability of a trait, there are several other research questions for which the twin study may have value. Differences in concordance rates between monozygotic and dizygotic twins may be investigated at the level of symptoms or symptom clusters to study the validity of symptom complexes. Varying forms or degrees of expression of a particular disease or trait in monozygotic twins may be a source of evidence of the validity of the construct or disease entity. The series of twin studies of population-based twin registries in the US, Australia, and Europe have yielded consistent findings regarding the importance of genetic etiology of many of the major psychiatric disorders, but also have begun to identify gene-environment interactions for some disorders such as depression (Kendler *et al.*, 1993; 1995; Wahlberg *et al.*, 1997).

Although current efforts in the field are now being placed on identifying DNA markers for psychiatric disorders, family and twin studies could still be employed to reduce the heterogeneity of current diagnostic classes and to enhance the validity of their definitions and subtypes thereof. One basic approach of genetic epidemiology is therefore to use within-family designs to minimize the probability of heterogeneity, assuming that the etiology of a disease is likely to be homotypic within families. This design reduces or eliminates the danger of genetic heterogeneity which is likely to characterize the psychiatric disorders, and it has important implications for the identification of specific genetic mechanisms of psychopathology.

***Adoption Studies***. Family and twin studies are genetically informative because they hold the environment 'constant' while examining the rates of disorder across different levels of genetic relationship. An alternative approach is to vary the environment while comparing individuals across degrees of genetic similarity. Adoption studies are part of this latter approach in that psychiatric similarity between an adoptee and his or her biological versus adoptive relatives is examined. An alternative design compares the biological relatives of affected adoptees with those of unaffected, or control adoptees. This approach is the most powerful for identifying genetic factors by minimizing the degree of familial aggregation that can be explained by same-environment confounds. However, adoption studies are also characterized by certain characteristics that may bias results. Biological parents of adopted children are known to have higher rates of psychopathology, alcoholism or criminality than other parents, and adopted children may themselves be at greater risk for psychiatric disorders (*e.g.* Bohman, 1978; Lipman, Offord, Boyle, & Racine, 1993). Although such criticisms may be valid reasons to carefully interpret the rates of disorder found in these studies, they do not negate the value of adoption studies to clarify genetic and environmental effects (in particular for disorders showing specificity of transmission). Estimates of heritability derived from adoption studies may also be used to examine the validity of different phenotypic definitions (Kety, Rosenthal, & Wender, 1968; Kendler, Gruenberg, and Kinney, 1984)

Perhaps the most powerful study design is the cross-fostering design in which offspring at risk for a particular disease are reared in the home of non-biologic parents with and without that disease. Through such a design, Tienari *et al.* (1994) recently provided evidence for gene-environment interaction in the etiology of schizophrenia.

***Biologic Markers in Relatives***. The most important strategy of relevance both to identification of the etiology of psychiatric disorders and to neuroscience is the high-risk design, which investigates unaffected offspring of parents with major psychiatric disorders compared to those of controls. Investigation of biologic markers within high-risk families is a powerful method to reduce the heterogeneity of unrelated samples, the strategy that has been traditionally employed in biologic psychiatry. For example, Friedman *et al.* (1988) have demonstrated a within-family link between schizophrenia spectrum and the N2 component of the event-related potential. By focusing on individuals with the greatest probability of developing specific disorders, the high risk design: a) maximizes the potential case yield; b) increases the power within the sample to observe hypothesized risk factor associations; c) increases the likelihood of observing the effects of mediating and moderating variables when drawing comparisons between and within subgroups of individuals with and without the primary risk factor (*e.g.* children of alcoholics with or without accompanying risk factors); and d) identifies early patterns of disease given the exposure (*e.g.* parental psychopathology).

Few of the high-risk studies to date, however, have studied the specificity of associations between vulnerability markers due to a lack of adequate controls. The inclusion of psychiatric comparison groups enables conclusions regarding the specificity of associations between a particular disorder and putative markers. For example, the results of our recent high risk study revealed different patterns of potentiated startle among offspring of parents with anxiety disorders compared to those of controls (Grillon *et al.*, 1997). Such studies will be increasingly important in studying the impact of genetic vulnerability factors and identifying environmental factors that may mediate genetic expression.

***Identification of Genes***. The rapid developments in molecular biology which have led to the identification of the primary gene defects for numerous diseases have proceeded far more slowly when applied to complex human disorders (such as the psychiatric disorders). Genes have generally been identified for diseases which are rare (*i.e.*, <.01% population prevalence), exhibit Mendelian patterns of inheritance, and can be clearly diagnosed with extremely high specificity and sensitivity (Risch, 1990). In contrast, the psychiatric disorders are complex disorders, which are conditions characterized by high population prevalence, a lack of clear distinction between affected and unaffected individuals (with the threshold for case definition being somewhat arbitrary) and failure to adhere to Mendelian patterns of transmission. Although recent progress in identification of the human gene map through the Human Genome Project and in development of statistical methods to assess complex models of transmission has enhanced the power of studies to identify the genetic basis of more complex diseases, linkage and association studies of common diseases with imprecise phenotypic definitions continue to be plagued by a lack of replication and inconsistent findings.

Inconclusive evidence regarding the role of genes in the etiology of the major psychiatric disorders can be attributed to their genetic complexity as well as to several other characteristics that have been identified through epidemiologic studies including: the high population prevalence; absence of diagnostic trait markers with high sensitivity and specificity; genetic and phenotypic heterogeneity; and gene-environment interaction.

***Psychiatric Disorder Phenotypes***. There is widespread agreement regarding the limitations in applying the current nomenclature for mental disorders to biologic studies. Psychiatric disorder phenotypes, based solely on clinical manifestations without pathognomonic markers, still lack conclusive evidence for validity of classification and reliability of measurement (Kendell, 1989). The lack of specificity of biologic and psychosocial risk factors and correlates, as well as the lack of longitudinal stability, still suggest etiologic and phenotypic heterogeneity.

The recent shift in psychiatric genetics to identify endophenotypes underlying biologic factors that explain familial recurrence is an important step in moving from broad phenotypes to specific components of disorders (Tsuang *et al.*, 1993) Recent advances in neuroscience and the behavioral sciences, not available to the pioneers in family study research in psychiatry, will be important tools in enhancing this process. Substantial effort should be devoted to the application of genetic epidemiologic studies that are designed to define more homogenous components of psychiatric disorders and associated biologic markers that may yield higher familial relative risk than the heterogeneous category of major depression.

Ironically, however, genetic mapping strategies may also assist in defining subtypes.

Nevertheless, lessons from other disorders have demonstrated that even after the identification of the gene for single gene disorders, the classification still requires additional testing to identify sources of heterogeneity in phenotypic expression. For example, despite the identification of the actual gene for Marfan's syndrome, the checklist criteria appear to be remarkably similar to those within the realm of DSM-IV (DePaepe *et al.*, 1996). Likewise, recent studies of neurofibromatosis have examined familial specificity of diverse clinical manifestations of the same genetic mutations.

***Lack of Direct Correspondence between the Genotype and Phenotype***. Application of advances in neuroscience and genetics to human diseases is still limited by the complexity of the process through which genes exert their influence. A lack of one-to-one correspondence between the genotype and phenotype is clearly the rule rather than the exception for most human disorders. Phenomena such as *penetrance* (*i.e.*, probability of phenotypic expression among individuals with susceptibility gene), v*ariable expressivity* (*i.e.*, degree to which susceptible individuals express components of genotype), *gene-environment interaction* (*i.e.*, expression of genotype only in presence of particular environmental exposures), *pleiotropy* (*i.e.*, capacity of gene to manifest simultaneously several different phenotypes), and *genetic heterogeneity* (*i.e.*, different genes leading to indistinguishable phenotypes) have been demonstrated for several human disorders for which susceptibility genes have been identified.

Breast cancer provides an illustration of *genetic heterogeneity*, another basic nosologic problem in genetics. Although family study research is beginning to examine differences in breast cancer among those with and without particular gene markers, the basic breast cancer phenotype has not been adequately differentiated. Patterns of comorbidity with other cancers and sex differences have been valuable in discriminating different genetic forms of breast cancer. Whereas families with predominantly affected females or those with both breast & ovarian cancer are more likely to have the BRCA1 mutation, families with male breast cancer primarily arise from the BRCA2 mutation (Ford *et al.*, 1994; Szabo & King, 1997). Thus, sex differences in recurrence risk and comorbidity across cancer types may be used to identify more homogeneous forms of cancer.

Breast cancer also provides an excellent illustration of the importance of community study data and epidemiologic approaches to risk estimation. Although the BRCA genes convey very high risk for the subsequent development of breast cancer at the level of the individual, their low population frequency diminishes the extent of breast cancer that is attributable to these genes. Hence, more than 90% of breast cancer cases are not attributable to mutations in these loci. Thus, in terms of public health significance, it is critical to identify other genetic and environmental risk factors that may explain the large number of nonBRCA cancer cases. The magnitude of ethnic/geographic heterogeneity which has been demonstrated for the BRCA gene and breast cancer also highlights the importance of epidemiologic data on the distribution of these polymorphisms in the general population (Szabo & King, 1997).

An integration of population genetics and epidemiology will be critical in determining the attributable risk of particular DNA markers for disease, the environmental conditions that potentiate or suppress expression of genetic vulnerability, and the implications of biologic and genetic markers for public health. Once these genes are identified for some of the major psychiatric disorders, genetic markers can be employed to gain understanding of their pathogenesis (Risch & Merikangas, 1996). Knowledge of trait markers may facilitate identification of the role of environmental factors, reduce the heterogeneity of the clinical phenotypes, inform psychiatric nosology, and permit more specific approaches to treatment and prevention of the major psychiatric conditions.

***Gene-environment interaction***. Gene-environment interaction characterizes a broad range of human diseases such as cancer and birth defects. The classic examples of gene-environment interaction are the inborn errors of metabolism, such as phenylketonuria, that manifest only when susceptible individuals are exposed to a particular protein or exogenous substance. Glucose-6-phosphate-dehydrogenase (G6PD) deficiency, an X-linked disorder caused by mutation on the long arm of the X chromosome, is another illustration of gene-environment interaction. The expression of this disorder becomes manifest as hemolytic anemia only when the susceptible individual is exposed to certain drugs or fava beans (Omenn & Motulsky, 1978). Birth defects have also been found to result from gene-environment interaction. For example, Hwang *et al.* (1997) assessed the effects of the interaction between maternal cigarette smoking and a transforming growth factor alpha (TGFA) polymorphism on the risk for oral clefts. Oral clefts were increased only among women with the TaqI polymorphism who smoked (Khoury). Likewise, many forms of cancer such as retinoblastoma (Vogel, 1979) arise from somatic mutations to the second allele among individuals who carry a susceptibility allele at a particular locus.

Not only is the expression of genes modified by the environment, but there is now substantial evidence to indicate that numerous environmental factors may actually alter the genotype as is characteristic of many forms of cancer. Francis and colleagues (1999) have shown that maternal behavior mediates stress reactivity in adulthood and is associated with future maternal behavior among offspring. Genes may also be involved in the response or resistance to purely environmental agents such as diet, stress, exercise, drugs, and nutritional deficiencies. The methods of genetic epidemiology are designed specifically to identify gene-environment interactions (Merikangas, in press).

## V11. Relevance of Epidemiology to Prevention

The ultimate goal of epidemiology is prevention of the incidence, progression and consequences of diseases. The traditional epidemiologic concept of the stages of prevention is comprised of three levels: (1) primary prevention which refers to measures that reduce the incidence of a disease; (2) secondary prevention which refers to measures that reduce the risk of disease among susceptible individuals; and (3) tertiary prevention which refers to efforts to reduce the impact or consequences of a disease.

At present, however, there is a major gap between prevention activities and empirical research. Following the now classic report of the Institute of Medicine Prevention Report (1994), and the National Mental Health Advisory Committee Work Group on Prevention (1999), there has been a large shift in the direction of prevention activity to incorporate the information gleaned from community-based research. A substantial proportion of prevention activity is not based on empirical data and is also of limited scope. With the increasingly discouraging results of many universal prevention trials, efforts are beginning to shift to employ the secondary rather than primary prevention. Both descriptive and analytic epidemiology will provide a valuable empirical basis for identifying targets and outcomes of such efforts.

There is an increasing awareness of the importance of populations, both in terms of understanding the etiology of disorders but also as the context for intervention (Weich, 1997). As the neurosciences continue to advance knowledge regarding human brain structure and function, the relevance of neurobiologic factors to mental disorders at the population level is likely to increase as we attempt to identify the extent to which basic sciences explain chronic human disease.

Advances in neuroscience, behavioral sciences and genetics are not only likely to enhance our understanding of the pathogenesis of mental disorders, but also to have major impact on treatment and prevention. Knowledge of trait markers will permit more specific approaches to treatment and prevention of the major psychiatric conditions. The relevance of advances in human genetics for prevention has been a somewhat controversial issue. Whereas some appropriate concern has been raised regarding the potential negative impact of identification of genetic risk factors in terms of stigma and misuse in reproductive planning, others envision the beneficial effects in preventing human disease and disability. Pre-diagnostic testing is now in widespread use for some well-characterized diseases. However, there is insufficient prognostic information for more complex disorders. Juengst *et al.* (1995) distinguished between phenotypic prevention and genotypic prevention. Whereas the former employs genetic information to prevent the clinical manifestations of susceptibility genes, the latter applies information on genotypes to prevent the transmission of the genes to subsequent generations through genetic counseling or pre-diagnostic testing.

One of the chief limitations of the application of risk research to prevention is the lack of a comprehensive understanding of the interactions among risk factors which may lead to disorders through a complex pattern of interactive influences. Moreover, many of the risk factors identified in epidemiologic research are fixed rather than malleable. Another important consideration in applying genetic risk factors to prevention concerns the low positive predictive value and population attributable fractions for most common chronic diseases (*e.g.* cholesterol and coronary heart disease) (Khoury, 1997). With advancing knowledge regarding both genetic risk factors, power to identify gene-environment interactions and ultimately to minimize exposure to environmental risk factors will provide the most important public health impact of genetic technology.

**FIGURE 1**
**Mental Health Intervention Spectrum**

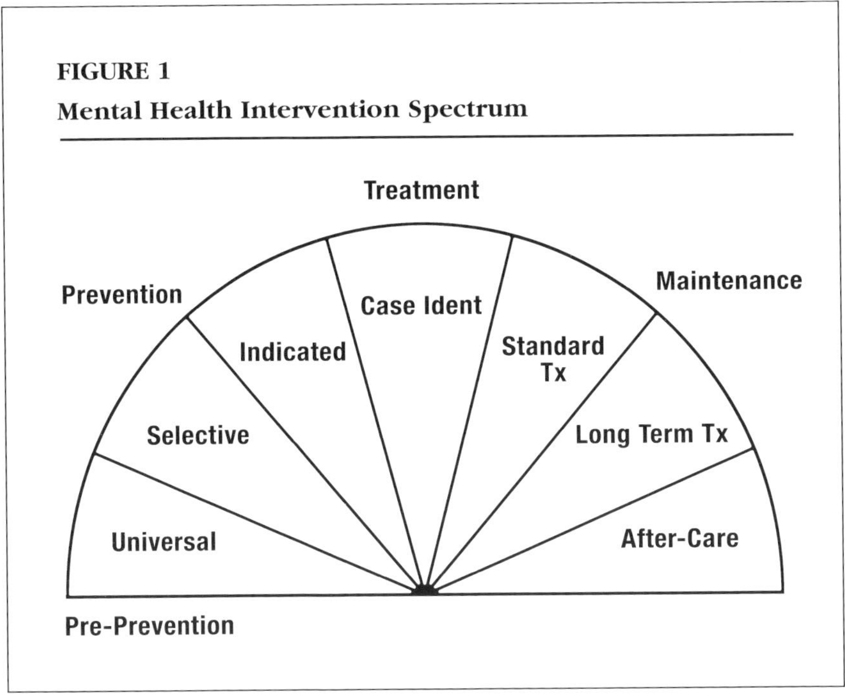


**Figure 1** depicts the Mental Health Intervention Spectrum first developed to describe the scope of prevention activities by the Institute of Medicine Prevention Committee (1995), and later adapted by the National Mental Health Advisory Council Work Group on Prevention Research (1999). The fluidity of the boundaries between different levels of prevention, particularly secondary and tertiary, is illustrated. Moreover there is a major shift in focus from primary prevention to secondary and tertiary efforts in minimizing recurrence and consequences as we apply this model to the mental disorders, most of which constitute chronic diseases. The Prevention Work Group introduced the concept of "pre-prevention" activities to depict the importance of research identifying targets and timing of prevention, as well as the relative public health significance of the major mental disorders.

One of the most promising prevention strategies is the primary prevention of secondary disorders described by Kessler and Frank (1996). This approach is most relevant to comorbid disorders in which one disorder is clearly a consequence of the primary disorder.

Family study research has demonstrated that the two major pathways to substance use disorders are social phobia and bipolar disorder (Merikangas *et al.*, 1998). A pilot study of prevention of substance abuse through application of cognitive behavioral therapy among adolescents with social anxiety disorder yielded promising results. (Dierker *et al.*, 2001). A larger intervention study in this pathway is now underway. Likewise, Geller *et al.* (1998) demonstrated that treatment of youth with both bipolar disorder and alcohol abuse or dependence led to diminution of both disorders.

## VIII. Summary

This paper has summarized the magnitude of the major mental disorders in adults and children in the U.S. Community study data reveal that approximately 20% of adults and children suffer from a mental disorder leading to significant impairment in their daily functioning. The burden and cost of these disorders is comparable to that of other major chronic diseases such as cardiovascular diseases and diabetes. Despite the disability resulting form these disorders, only a minority receive treatment. The subjective anguish resulting from these disorders is immeasurable.

There is widespread agreement regarding the limitations in applying the current nomenclature for mental disorders to etiologic studies. Mental disorder phenotypes, based solely on clinical manifestation without pathognomonic markers, still lack conclusive evidence for validity of classification and reliability of measurement. The lack of specificity of biologic and psychosocial risk factors and correlates, as well as the lack of longitudinal stability still suggest etiologic and phenotypic heterogeneity. Current evidence favors multifactorial etiology of the major mental disorders, which result from mutually interactive influences of genetic, biologic and contextual risk factors.

The familial recurrence risks are significantly elevated for all of the major mental disorders, irrespective of the sampling and methods employed. The risk ratios are greatest for bipolar disorder and schizophrenia ranging from 6-10, intermediate for substance dependence (average 4-8) and subtypes of anxiety, particularly panic (*i.e.* 5%) and lowest for major depression (*i.e.* average of 2-3). The lack of conclusive evidence regarding the role of genes in the etiology of the major psychiatric disorders can be attributed to their genetic complexity as reflected by gene-environment interaction, genetic and phenotypic heterogeneity, and limitations in the validity of diagnostic classification. The recent shift in psychiatric genetics to identify endophenotypes, underlying biologic factors that explain familial recurrence, is an important step in moving from broad phenotypes to specific components of disorders. Recent advances in neuroscience and the behavioral sciences, not available to the pioneers in family study research in psychiatry, will be important tools in enhancing this process.

There is also an increasing awareness of the importance of populations as the context for intervention (Weich, 1997). As the neurosciences continue to advance knowledge regarding human brain structure and function, the relevance of neurobiologic factors to psychiatric disorders at the population level is likely to increase as we attempt to identify the extent to which basic sciences explain chronic human disease.

## References


American Psychiatric Association (1994). Diagnostic and Statistical Manual of Mental Disorders (4th edition) (DSM-IV). Washington, D.C.: APA.

Anderson, J., Williams, S., McGee, R., & Silva, P. (1987). DSM-III disorders in preadolescent children. *Archives of General Psychiatry*, 44: 69-76.

Angst, J. & Merikangas, K. (1997). The depressive spectrum: diagnostic classification and course. *Journal of Affective Disorders*. 45: 31-39.

Angst. J., Merikangas K.R., Preisig M. (1997). Subthreshold syndromes of depression and anxiety in the community. *J Clin Psychiatry*, 58: 6-10.

Bird, H.R., Canino, G., Rubio-Stipec, M., & Gould, M.S. (1988). Estimates of prevalence of childhood maladjustment in a community survey in Puerto Rico, *Archives of General Psychiatry*, 45: 1120-1126.

Boyle, M.H., Offord, D.R., Hofman, H.G. , Catlin, G.P. Byles, J.A. Cadman, D.T., Crawford, J.W., Links, P.S., Rae-Grant, N.I., & Szatmari, P. (1987). Ontario Child Health Study I. *Archives of General Psychiatry* 44: 826-831.

Bromet, E.J., Dew, M.A., & Eaton, W. (1995). Epidemiology of psychosis with special reference to schizophrenia. In M.T. Tsuang, M. Tohen, & G.E.P. Zahner (Eds.) Textbook in Psychiatric Epidemiology. Wiley-Liss: New York. 283-300.

Brown, G.W., Harris, T. (1978) The Social Origins of Depression: A Study of Psychiatric Disorder in Women. London: Tavistock.

Child, A.H. (1997).Marfan syndrome—current medical and genetic knowledge: How to treat and when. *J Card Surg*, 12 (Suppl 2): 131-136.

Cohen, P., & Brook, J. (1987). Family factors related to the persistence of psychopathology in childhood and adolescents. *Psychiatry*, 50: 332-345.

Costello, E.J. (1989). Developments in child psychiatric epidemiology. *Journal of the American Academy of Child and Adolescent Psychiatry*, 28: 836-841.

Costello, E.J., Costello, A.J., Edelbrock, C., Burns, B., Dulcan, M., Brent, D., & Janiszewski, S. (1988). Psychiatric disorders in pediatric primary care: Prevalence and risk factors. *Archives of General Psychiatry*, 45: 1107-1116.

De Paepe, A., Devereoux, T.B., Dietz, H.C., Hennekam, R.C., Pyeritz, R.E.: Revised diagnostic criteria for Marfan Syndrome. *Am J Med Genet* 62:417-426, 1996.

Dierker, L., Albano, A., Clarke, G., Heimberg, R., Kendall P., Merikangas, K., Lewinsohn, P., Offord, D., Kessler, R., Kupfer, D. Screening for anxiety and depression in early adolescence. *J American Academy of Child and Adolescent Psychiatry* (2001). 40:929-936.

Endicott, J., Spitzer, R.L. (1978). A diagnostic interview: The schedule for affective disorders and schizophrenia. *Archives of General Psychiatry* 35:837-844.

Feighner, J.P., Robins, E., Guze, S.B., Woodruff, R.A., Winokur, G., & Munoz, R. (1972). Diagnostic criteria for psychiatric research. *Archives of General Psychiatry* 16: 57-63.

Ford, D., Easton, D.F., Bishop, D.T., *et al*: (1994) Risks of cancer in BRCA1-mutation carriers. Breast Cancer Linkage Consortium. *Am J Hum Genet* 56: 265-71.

Francis, D., Diorio, J., Liu, D., Meaney, M.J. (1999) Nongenomic transmission across generations of maternal behavior and stress responses in the rat. *Science*, 286: 1155-1158.

Friedman, R., Katz-Leavy, J., Manderscheid, R., & Sondheimer, D. (1996a). Prevalence of serious emotional disturbance in children and adolescents. In R. W. Manderscheid & M. A. Sonnenschein (Eds.), Mental health, United States, 1996 (pp. 77-91). Washington, DC: U.S. Government Printing Office.

Friedman, D., Cornblatt, B., Vaughan, H., & Erlenmeyer-Kimling, L. (1988). Auditory eventrelated potentials in children at risk for schizophrenia: The complete initial sample. *Psychiatry Research*, 26, 203-221.

Garmezy, N. (1983). Stressors of childhood. In N. Garmezy & M. Rutter (Eds.), Stress, Coping, and Development in Children (pp. 43-84). New York: McGraw-Hill.

Garvey, M. A., Giedd, J., & Swedo, S. E. (1998). PANDAS: The search for environmental triggers of pediatric neuropsychiatric disorders. Lessons from rheumatic fever. *Journal of Child Neurology*, 13: 413-423.

Geller, B., Cooper, T. B., Sun, K., Zimmerman, B., Frazier, J., Williams, M., & Heath, J. (1998). Double-blind and placebo-controlled study of lithium for adolescent bipolar disorders with secondary substance dependency. *Journal of the American Academy of Child and Adolescent Psychiatry*, 37: 171-178.

Grillon, C., Dierker, L., & Merikangas, K.R. (1997). Startle modulation in children at risk for anxiety disorders and/or alcoholism. *Journal of the American Academy of Child and Adolescent Psychiatry*, 36: 925-932.

Institute of Medicine. (1994). Reducing Risks for Mental Disorders: Frontiers for Preventive Intervention Research. Washington, DC: National Academy Press.

Hafner, H., Riecher-Rossler, A., An Der Heiden, W., Maurer, K., Fatkenheuer B., & Loffler, W. (1993). Generating and testing a causal explanation of the gender difference in age at first onset of schizophrenia. *Psychological Medicine*, 23: 925-940.

Hall, J.M., Lee, M.K., Morrow, J., Newman, B., Anderson, L., Huey, B., & King, M.C. (1990). Linkage analysis of early onset familial breast cancer to chromosome 17q21. *Science*, 250: 1684-1689.

Henderson, A.S. (1996). The present state of psychiatric epidemiology. *Australia and New Zealand Journal of Psychiatry*, 30: 9-19.

Hill, S.Y., Neiswanger, K. (1997). The Value of Narrow Psychiatric Phenotypes and "Super" Normal Controls. New York: CRC Press.

Hwang, S.J., Beaty, T.H., Panny, S.R., (1995), Association study of transforming growth factor alpha TaqI polymorphisms and oral clefts: Indication of gene-environment interaction in a population-based sample of infants with birth defects. *American Journal of Epidemiology*, 141: 629-636

Juengst, E. (1995). Prevention and the goals of genetic medicine. *Human Gene Therapy*, 6: 835-844.

Khoury, M. (1997). Relationship between medical genetics and public health: Changing the paradigm of disease prevention and the definition of a genetic disease. *American Journal of Medical Genetics*, 71: 289-291.

Kendell, R.E. (1989). Clinical validity. *Psychological Medicine*, 19: 45-55.

Kendler, K.S. (1995). Genetic epidemiology in psychiatry: Taking both genes and environment seriously. *Archives of General Psychiatry*, 52: 895-899.

Kendler, K.S. (1990). The super-normal control group in psychiatric genetics: Post artifactual evidence for aggregation. *Psychiatric Genetics*; 1:45-53

Kendler, K.S., Neale, M.C., Kessler, R.C., Heath A.C., Eaves, L.J.; (1992). A population-based twin study of major depression in women: The impact of varying definitions of illness. *Archives of General Psychiatry* 49: 257-266.

Kendler, K.S., Neale, M.C., Kessler, R.C., Heath, A.C., & Eaves, L.J. (1993). Major depression and phobias: The genetic and environmental sources of comorbidity. *Psychological Medicine*, 23: 361-371.

Kessler R. (1999). The World Health Organization International Consortium in Psychiatric Epidemiology (ICPE): initial work and future directions-the NAPE Lecture. *Acta Psychiatrica Scandinavica*; 99: 2-9.

Kessler, R.C., McGonagle, K.A., Zhao, S., Nelson, C.B., Hughes, M., Eshleman, S., Wittchen, H.U., & Kendler, K. S. (1994). Lifetime and 12-month prevalence of DSM-Hl-R psychiatric disorders in the United States. *Archives of General Psychiatry* 51; 8-19.

Kessler, R. C., Nelson, M. B., McGonagle, K. A., & Edlund, M. J. (1996). The epidemiology of co-occurring mental disorders and substance use disorders in the National Comorbidity Study: implications for prevention and service utilization. *American Journal of Orthopsychiatry*, 66: 17-31.

Kety, S.S., Rosenthal, D., & Wender, P.H. (1968). The types and prevalence of mental illness in the biological and adoptive families of adopted schizophrenics. In The Transmission of Schizophrenia. D. Rosenthal & S. Kety (Eds). London: Pergamon.

Khoury, M. (1997a). Genetic epidemiology and the future of disease prevention and public health. *Epidemiologic Reviews,* 19: 175.

Khoury M. (1997b). Relationship between medical genetics and public health: Changing the paradigm of disease prevention and the definition of a genetic disease. *American Journal of Medical Genetics*, 71: 289-291.

Khoury, M.J., Dorman, J.S. (1998). The Human Genome Epidemiology Network. *American Journal of Epidemiology* 1998; 148: 1-3.

Kleinbaum, D.G., Kupper, L.L., & Morgenstern, H. (1982). Epidemiologic research: Principles and quantatative methods. Belmont, California: Wadsworth.

Kuller, L.H. (1979). The role of population genetics in the study of the epidemiology of cardiovascular risk factors, In Genetics analysis of common diseases: Applications to predictive factors in coronary disease. New York: Liss.

Loeber, R. (1991). "Antisocial Behavior: More enduring than changeable?" *Journal of the American Academy of Child and Adolescent Psychiatry* 30: 393-397.

Mausner, J.S., & Baun, A.K. (1984). Epidemiology: an Introductory Text. Philadelphia: WB Saunders.

Merikangas, K.R.: (1999). Editorial: The next decade of psychiatric epidemiology. *International Journal of Methods in Psychiatric Research* 8:1-5, 1999

Merikangas, K.R. Genetic epidemiology: Bringing genetics to the population. *Acta Psychiatrica Scandinavica*, in press.

Merikangas, K.R., Angst, J., Eaton, W., Canino, G., Rubio-Stipec, M., Wacker, H. *et al.* (1996). Comorbidity and boundaries of affective disorders with anxiety disorders and substance misuse: Results of an international task force. *British Journal of Psychiatry* 168 (suppl 30): 58-67.

Merikangas, K.R., Angst, J. (1996). The challenge of depressive disorders in adolescence. In Rutter (Ed.) Psychosocial disturbances in young people: Challenges for prevention. New York: Cambridge University Press. p.131, p.165.

Merikangas, K.R., Swendsen, J. (1997). The genetic epidemiology of psychiatric disorders. *Epidemiologic Reviews.* p.19, pp.1-12.

Merikangas, K.R., Mehta, R.I., Molnar, B.E. *et al.* (1998). Comorbidity of substance use disorders with mood and anxiety disorders: Results of the International Consortium in Psychiatric Epidemiology. *Addictive Behavior* 23: 893-907.

Morton, N.E. (1982). Outline of genetic epidemiology. Basel: Karger.

Murray, C.J.L., Lopez A.D., eds. (1996). The Global Burden of Disease and Injury Series, Volume 1. A comprehensive assessment of mortality and disability from diseases, injuries and risk factors in 1990 and projected to 2020. Cambridge, MA: Harvard School of Public Health on behalf of the World Health Organization and the World Bank; Harvard University Press.

Offord, D.R., Boyle, M.H., Szatmari, P., Rae-Grant, N., Links, P.S., Cadman, D.T., Byles, J.A. Crawford, J.W., Blum, H.M., Byrne, C., Thomas, H., & Woodward, C.A.(1987). Ontario Child Health Study II. Six month prevalence rates and service utilization. *Archives of General Psychiatry*, 44: 832-836.

Omenn, G.S., Motulsky, A.G. (1978). Ecogenetics: Genetic variation in susceptibility to environmental agents. In: Cohen BH, Lilienfeld AM, Huang PC, editors. Genetic issues in public health and medicine. Springfield: Thomas; 1978. p. 83-111.

Orvaschel, H., Puig-Antich, J., Chambers, W., Tabrizi, M. A., & Johnson, R. (1982). Retrospective assessment of prepubertal major depression with the Kiddie-SADS-E. *Journal of the American Academy of Child Psychiatry*, 21: 392-397.

Peltonen, L., McKusick VA. (2001). Dissecting human disease in the postgenomic era. *Science*, 291: 1224-1228.

Regier, D.A., Burke, J.D., & Burke, K.C.(1990). Comorbidity of affective and anxiety disorders in the NIMH epidemiologic catchment area (ECA) program. Comorbidity of Mood and Anxiety Disorders. J. D. Maser and C. R. Cloninger. Washington D.C.: American Psychiatric Press, Inc.: pp.113-122.

Reus, V.I., Freimer, N.B. Behavioral Genetics '97. (1997). Understanding the genetic basis of mood disorders: Where do we stand? *American Journal of Human Genetics*; 60: 1283-1288.

Risch, N. (1990). Linkage strategies for genetically complex traits. I. Multilocus models. *American Journal of Human Genetics*, 46: 222-228.

Risch, N. (1994). Mapping genes for psychiatric disorders. In E.S. Gershon, & C.R. Cloninger (Eds.) Genetic approaches to mental disorders. Washington, D.C.: American Psychiatric Press. pp.47-61.

Risch, N., (2000a). Searching for genes in complex diseases: lessons from systemic lupus erythematosus *The Journal of Clinical Investigation*. 105: 503-1506.

Risch N. (2000). Searching for genetic determinants in the new millennium. *Nature*, 405: 847-856.

Risch, N., & Merikangas, K.R. (1996). The future of genetic studies of complex human diseases. *Science*, 273: 1516-1517.

Robins, L. (1992). The future of psychiatric epidemiology. *International Journal of Methods in Psychiatric Research*, 2: 1-3.

Robins, L., Helzer J, Croughan J, Ratcliff KS (1981). The NIMH Diagnostic Interview Schedule: Its history, characteristics and validity. *Archives of General Psychiatry*, 45: 381-389.

Robins, L.N., Wing, J.K., Wittchen, H.U., Helzer, J.E., Babor, T.F., Burke, J., Farmer, A., Jablenski, A., Pickens, R., Regier, D.A. Sartorius, N., Towle, L.H. (1988). The Composite International Diagnostic Interview. *Archives of General Psychiatry* 45: 1069-1077.

Rutter, M. (1989). Isle of Wight revisited: Twenty-five years of child psychiatric epidemiology. *Journal of the American Academy of Child and Adolescent Psychiatry* 28: 633-653.

Spitzer, R.L., William, J.B., Gibbon, M., First, M.B. (1992). The Sturctured Clinical Interview for DSM-III-R (SCID). I. History, rationale and description. *Archives of General Psychiatry* 49: 624-629.

Szabo, C., & King, M.C. (1997). Population genetics of BRCA1 and BRCA2. *American Journal of Human Genetics*, 60: 1013-1020.

Tienari, P., Wynne, L.C., Moring, J., Lahti, I., Naarala, M., Sorri, A., Wahlberg, K.E., Saarento, O., Seitamaa, M., Kaleva, M., *et al.* (1994) The Finnish adoptive family study of schizophrenia: implications for family research. *British Journal of Psychiatry*; 23:20-6.

Tsuang, M.T., Faraone, S.V., Lyons, M.J. (1993). Identification of the phenotype in psychiatric genetics. *European Archives of Psychiatry and Clinical Neuroscience*, 243: 131-42.

U.S. Department of Health and Human Services. Mental Health: A Report of the Surgeon General-Executive Summary. Rockville, MD: US Department of Health and Human Services, Substance Abuse and Mental Health Services Administration, Center for Mental Health Services, National Institutes of Health, National Institute of Mental Health, 1999.

Vogel F. (1979). Genetics of retinoblastoma. *Human Genetics*, 52: 1-54.

Vogel, F., Motulsky, A.G. (1995). Human Genetics: Problems and Approaches. 3rd ed. Berlin: Springer Verlag.

Wahlberg, K.E., Wynne, L.C., Oja, H., Keskitalo, P., Pykalainen., L., Lahti, I., Moring, J., Naarala, M., Sorri, A., Seitamaa, M., Laksy, K., Kolassa, J., & Tienari, P. (1997). Gene-environment interaction in vulnerability to schizophrenia: findings from the Finnish Adoptive Family Study of Schizophrenia. *American Journal of Psychiatry*, 154: 355-362.

Weich, S. (1997) Prevention of the common mental disorders. *Psychological Medicine*, 27: 757-764.

Weissman, M.M. (1996). Cross-national epidemiology of depression and bipolar disorder. *JAMA*. 276: 293-299.

Whittemore, A. (1999). The Eighth AACR American Cancer Society Award lecture on cancer epidemiology and prevention. Genetically tailored preventive strategies: an effective plan for the twenty-first century? American Association for Cancer Research. *Cancer Epidemiology, Biomarkers & Prevention* 8: 649-658.

Wing, J.K., Cooper, J.E., & Sartorius, N. (1974). Measurement and Classification of Psychiatric Symptoms: An Instructional Manual for the PSE and CATEGO Program. New York, Cambridge University Press. World Health Organization (1993).

Yang, Q., Khoury, M.J. (1997). Evolving methods in genetic epidemiology III. Gene-environment interaction in epidemiologic research. *Epidemiologic Reviews*, 19: 33-43.

## Improving Access to Evidence-Based Services: Translating Need into Supply and Demand

**Howard H. Goldman, M.D., Ph.D.**
**University of Maryland School of Medicine**

*Mental Health - A Report of the Surgeon General* provides a comprehensive look at mental health from a public health perspective. The landmark report reviews 3000 scientific papers and draws upon the expertise of dozens of contributors. It details information on mental disorders and their treatment and it describes the service system supporting those treatments. No single aspect of the report has created so much attention, however, as the evidence of the magnitude of the problem. From a public health perspective the prevalence of mental disorders and the associated disability are critical factors. One-in-five individuals experiences one of a specific list of mental disorders in the course of any given year; and that climbs to one-in-four, if we include substance abuse disorder. The *Global Burden of Disease* report indicates that the mental disorders account for more than 15% of the overall burden of disease from *all* causes. This is about the same level of burden as cancer and just trails all cardiovascular conditions, the leading cause of disability worldwide, accounting for 18% of the global burden. The public health alarm, however, is caused by the observation that only about one-in-three of such individuals receives any treatment during the course of the year.

No single aspect of the report also generated so much controversy. Although the data demonstrating the prevalence of mental disorders are consistent and several decades old and newer data sustain the magnitude of the problem, critics question the validity of mental disorders and the methods used to define and identify them. To disbelievers the one-in-five prevalence figure is preposterously high. Critics deride the *Diagnostic and Statistical Manual of Mental Disorders* of the American Psychiatric Association as an arbitrary compendium reflecting a nosology determined by a vote of self-interested experts. They criticize the lack of lesions to define the conditions, the use of menus of symptoms to define disorders, and the vague boundaries between normal and abnormal behavior. They are not surprised by the finding that only one-in-three individuals who meet the criteria for a mental disorder seek care. They argue that perhaps that is more than the appropriate level for conditions that may not *need* treatment. They also point out that an equal number of individuals *do* seek care even though they do not meet the criteria for one of the listed mental disorders. The report explains that the list is not all-inclusive, that many of the individuals who used services had just one-too-few symptoms to meet the specified criteria — or that they had a mental disorder in the immediate past. The report also explains that many of the data on prevalence do not get to the heart of "clinical significance," and that perhaps only about one-in-ten individuals has a clinically significant condition. This interpretation would close the gap between need and use, but the gap remains a public health problem all the same.

The fact remains, however, that current science does not provide a very good measure of the *need* for treatment or for mental health services. We continue to infer need from prevalence or better yet from measures of dysfunction and disability. Often we are left to use data on use of services as a proxy for need. We infer need from use and from *demand* for service — the economic perspective on use in the face of a price in a market, given a particular level of supply of treatment services.

*The Report of the Surgeon General* also addresses another powerful criticism of the mental health field. Skeptics about the validity of mental disorders continue their opposition to concerns about mental health with a critique of treatment. Even when critics concede that there are mental disorders or that some individuals experience mental distress and dysfunction, they question the effectiveness of treatment. If there are no effective treatments available, why be concerned about barriers to help-seeking behavior? Some critics even argue that the stigma associated with mental disorder is a *good* thing, reducing the demand for an expensive and wasteful service. The main finding of the report, however, cuts the feet out from under these skeptics when it concludes: *The efficacy of a range of treatments for most mental disorders is well documented.* This finding reinforces the societal benefit associated with help-seeking behavior if it results in provision and receipt of evidence-based services. The gap between the need for treatment and the demand for treatment is important because it means that individuals are not able to benefit from effective treatment. The global burden of disease associated with mental illness remains high when effective treatments and services are not used.

This paper explores the relationship among the need for treatment, the demand for services, and the supply of individuals and programs capable of providing needed and effective treatment to the population. The disparity between the opportunities afforded by advances in treatment and the reality of practice represents a significant public health challenge to the nation and the world at large. The 2001 World Health Report from the World Health Organization is devoted to mental health and speaks to the global nature of this problem. This paper focuses on implementing evidence-based practices to address the disparity between opportunity and reality, after establishing a conceptual framework and reviewing what we know about need, demand, and supply. The paper concludes with a review of the specific courses of action outlined by the Surgeon General to implement evidence-based practices:

- Continue to develop the science base
- Overcome stigma
- Improve awareness of effective treatment
- Ensure the supply of mental health services and providers
- Ensure delivery of state-of-the-art treatments
- Tailor treatment to age, gender, race, and culture
- Facilitate entry into treatment
- Reduce financial barriers to treatment

The main focus of the conference is on the fourth of the courses of action presented by the Surgeon General — ensure the supply of mental health services and providers. This paper places that single course of action in the broader context of all of the other courses of action and the economic and social organizational forces shaping the current context of mental health services delivery. It will argue that the workforce problem is but one manifestation of a larger problem of creating the proper incentives to implement evidence-base practices. The paper's perspective is taken from health services research and economics, informed by current experiences with efforts to implement evidence-based practices with the existing workforce. It should also inform efforts to train a new workforce of yet-to-be-trained professionals. It begins with several models for looking at implementing evidence-based practices - rooted both in the literature on technology transfer and in political economics.

### Implementing Evidence-Based Practices – Modeling the Process

The conventional process for determining workforce needs in health care is exemplified by the rational planning model of the Graduate

Medical Education National Advisory Council [GMENAC]. GMENAC projected needs for various health care providers after an elaborate process of determining treatment and service needs for individuals with specific health conditions. They calculated how much service was required and what personnel were required to deliver the care and treatment. Current workforce levels would be compared with data of the number of trainees in the "pipeline" and estimates were provided for future workforce requirements. The process generated overall and regional workforce estimates. The accuracy of the process depends on the ability to estimate need with accuracy and to translate population-based needs into specific treatment and related workforce requirements. There have been ongoing efforts to improve the information available to drive such a process, but imperfect information has yielded imperfect and highly disputed estimates. Workforce, training, and education planning and policy making have not been rational processes driven by information. They do not occur in a vacuum but are subject to the forces within the political economy, influenced by regional politics, academic pork-barreling, professional associations, specialty societies, consumer pressures and various disease-specific lobbying. All of these forces distort the rational planning as much as the lack of information to drive GMENAC-type models.

This paper has already suggested that our concepts and information on estimating needs are deficient. Further we have indicated that current practice, often the basis for workforce estimates, is not evidence-based practice. It would not do to estimate workforce demands on the basis of "usual care" as this would mis-specify what is truly required of a workforce for the future – at least a workforce best able to deliver effective services and meet the treatment needs of the population. It would be possible to replicate the GMENAC estimates of the past, but to do so would ignore the larger context and the greater challenge. The problem of "educating health professionals to meet new needs" begins with the problem of implementing evidence-based practices more broadly. This paper re-frames the issue to focus on implementing evidence-based practices. It conceptualizes the problem as one of getting professionals to use evidence-based practices routinely, where available. This leaves plenty of room for clinical judgment - evidence is imperfect and incomplete - but it focuses on the current training and practice needs for current professionals and for professionals in training.

The topic of "evidence-based practice" sometimes engenders very defensive responses from practicing clinicians and from the general population alike. "What do we practice [receive] now, if not evidence-based practice?" Unfortunately the data on practice and adherence to guidelines and standards of practice suggests otherwise. The Institute of Medicine recently focused attention on the "quality chasm" and various studies on unexplained regional practice variations testify to the gap between evidence-based practices and usual care. Specific studies have documented this type of problem in mental health practice - for example in the treatment of depression and schizophrenia. *The Report of the Surgeon General* offers some illustrations of the problem and identifies closing this gap as a critical issue for mental health care. Ironically as scientific advances increase the call for implementing evidence-based practices, the field has little data to guide such implementation. We are on our own without much evidence with our efforts to implement such practices. Most of the empirical research has told us that conventional educational techniques do not work and are not the answer to quality improvement. Exploratory research has led to several theoretical models to guide the next generation of implementation evaluations, but the research has not provided much more than a list of obvious "do's and don'ts."

One of the most popular models comes from the work of Green. This model emphasizes three key elements of the implementation process: 1) predisposing or disseminating strategies [*e.g.* training interventions and materials], 2) enabling methods [*e.g.* practice guidelines and supervision], and 3) reinforcing strategies [*e.g.* practice feedback]. These elements can be important at various levels of social organization – a clinical practice, an agency or facility, a local health or mental health authority, or a state authority. Furthermore, the model suggests that interventions to implement evidence-based practices should be directed to patients and clients themselves and to their families.

The recognition of the multiplicity of actors in the implementation process and the limitations of previous models to explain behavior led our research center's "dissemination core" to conceptualize this area of investigation as an inquiry in political economics. Implementation directed at patients/clients and their families, designed to "activate" them as "informed consumers," is conceptualized as *demand-side* intervention. Like direct-to-consumer advertising, demand-side interventions are intended to inform consumers of the benefits of evidence-based practices so that they will request them from clinicians and clinical programs. Traditional dissemination and training activity designed to directly shape the practice behavior of providers is conceptualized as *supply-side* intervention. There are newer techniques for changing practices, such as "academic detailing," a process that borrows the persuasive methods of the pharmaceutical sales force and couples them with the evidence-based practices of the "academy." Third are the regulatory interventions that alter practices by creating financial and organizational incentives to encourage evidence-based practices. These *regulatory* interventions include changes in insurance coverage policy to favor evidence-based practices or organizational strategies to permit new practices to be undertaken (*e.g.* licensure policies or adding medications to formularies).

Whatever conceptual model might prove to be best at understanding the process of implementing evidence-based practices, more information is needed about the basic elements of health service delivery – need, demand, supply, and financing - particularly in the current managed care environment.

## What Do We Actually Know About Demand for Services?

According to estimates prepared for the *The Report of the Surgeon General* from several national sources, about 20% of the U.S. population are affected by a mental disorder during the course of the year. The prevalence estimate is similar for children and adolescents, adults, and older adults, although the list of specific disorders for each age group is different and the distribution of conditions varies. In addition, about 3% of the adult population have a co-occurring substance abuse disorder and 6% have an addictive disorder alone. As noted earlier, these estimates focus on diagnostic criteria based on patterns of symptoms that occur together for specified time periods. Not all of these disorders are thought to be "clinically significant" and requiring treatment. Using functional criteria, it is estimated that about 9% of all adults in the U.S. have one of the mental disorders included in the national prevalence estimates and experience significant functional impairment. About 5% of the adult population are considered to have a "serious" mental illness and half of them have a "severe and persistent" mental illness. Social Security provides disability benefits to approximately 0.5% of the adult population. The report then goes on to explain the difficulty in identifying a "case" of mental disorder and in establishing the need for treatment.

The concern about a precise definition of a "case" and the deficiencies in assessing need for treatment become issues when considering utilization and demand for services. Approximately 15% of the population seek treatment services for a mental disorder each year. Although only about 8% of the population both have a diagnosis and receive treatment, about 7% receive treatment but do not meet diagnostic criteria for a mental disorder. Most of those who do not have a current diagnosis previously had a diagnosis or have a condition that just misses meeting diagnostic criteria. They appear to have some level of distress and/or dysfunction to cause them to seek treatment services. What is the right prevalence figure to use when estimating need and determining un-met need? When the Surgeon General expresses concern that only one-third of individuals with a mental disorder seeks mental health care this must be seen in the context of the limitations of our surveillance techniques and our definitions of need. If functional criteria identify those in need, then the 9% prevalence figure [for those meeting diagnostic criteria and demonstrating functional impairment] is matched pretty closely by a figure of 8% utilization. Yet the data indicate that there is a population at some level of need who do not meet diagnostic criteria for a mental disorder but experience some degree of distress and functional impairment. Surely there are more people "in need" than served currently in either the specialty or general medical and social welfare sectors — but just how many is not clear.

Ambiguities about need shift the focus in most mental health services research to studies of patterns of use and demand in specific populations under specific economic conditions [*e.g.* income and insurance coverage]. Demand is an economic concept used for studying utilization and cost of services. Typically demand is viewed in two components: *probability of use* and *quantity of use*. Probability of use is defined by the proportion of individuals in a population who use *any* service; quantity of use measures the *amount* of services used. Probability of use provides one indicator of access to care; quantity of use in monetary terms tells us about *expenditures*. Focusing on specific sub-populations and their economic circumstances [such as insurance coverage] reveals the heterogeneity of the population, obscured by national data. Although 15% of the population may use any mental health service during the course of the year, the treated prevalence rates vary greatly from group to group, depending on their socioeconomic characteristics and the state of their insurance coverage and the degree of managed care they experience. Utilization rates are comparatively high for Medicaid populations and individuals in state mental health systems; probability of use may be as low as one percent in some employer-based, insured sub-populations in health maintenance organizations, for example. It is hard to identify the "right" level of use, when it is so difficult to estimate need, but these data are at the heart of discussions of policy.

Estimating workforce requirements from data on need, prevalence, and demand is difficult, given the imperfections of the science. Furthermore, using data on existing patterns of care and existing practices in "usual care" will not tell us what individuals *should* be receiving care and from whom. It also will not tell us how to train the workforce and re-train current practitioners. Only by attending to evidence-based practices can this more sensible objective be achieved. Before examining these more basic questions related to evidence-based services, the paper examines what is known about where care currently is provided and by whom.

**What Do We Actually Know About the Supply of Providers?**

The 15% of adults who use any mental health service do so in a variety of settings. About 11% of them receive services in the health sector, almost equally divided between specialty providers [such as psychiatric hospitals and clinics] and general medical providers [such as primary care doctors]. These 11% overlap to some extent with 5% of the population who receive mental health services from other human service providers [such as social services and school-based counseling] and 3% who obtain care in the voluntary support network of self-help groups and peer counseling. Of the 21% of children and adolescents who use mental health services, 9% use health services [8% in specialty services overlapping with 3% in general medical care]. Seventeen percent receive their care [with substantial overlap with health care] from other human service professionals, almost entirely from the school system. This diversity of settings for care suggests the variety of individual providers, professional and para-professional, who constitute the mental health care workforce, delivering care and treatment to individuals with mental health problems.

The federal Center for Mental Health Services published Mental Health, United States, 1998 with an entire chapter devoted to providing data on "Mental Health Practitioners and Trainees." The volume tracks changes between 1982 and 1998 in the supply of clinically trained mental health personnel in 8 disciplines: psychiatry, psychology, social work, psychiatric nursing, counseling, marriage and family therapy, psychosocial rehabilitation, and school psychology. The data reflect the diversity and growth of mental health professionals. The volume also presents data on the demographic characteristics of the workforce. Nowhere is there a comprehensive picture of what these personnel are doing. How many are trained in evidence-based psychotherapies? Who among the psychiatrists are skilled in the use of newer psychotropic agents? How many have experience working with individuals with mental and addictive disorders in integrated treatment? Although it is important to know how many and what kinds professionals we have, knowing what they do and what they need to do is central to the task of projecting the workforce needs for the immediate and longer-term future.

### What Do We Actually Know About the Supply of Evidence-Based Services?

A growing literature documents the inappropriate variations and quality deficiencies of typical health and mental health practice. As noted above, advances in the scientific basis for treatment and services make these variations and deficiencies a serious public health problem. The mental health report of the Surgeon General summarized two areas where these quality problems recently have been identified - in the treatment of depression, particularly in primary care settings, and in the care and treatment of schizophrenia. In primary care settings, for example, one-third to one-half of patients with major depression are not recognized as being depressed. Poor care results from under-recognition, and when depression is recognized, often it is inappropriately treated. Medication frequently is discontinued before achieving a good clinical result, and effective psychotherapies are not recommended. Even when psychotherapy is recommended, it is difficult to find a practitioner skilled in one of the evidence-based therapies. Primary care doctors are not trained to deliver such services and referrals are not available. The story is similar for the specialty care and treatment of schizophrenia. That was the conclusion of the Schizophrenia Patient Outcome Research Team study, conducted at the University of Maryland and Johns Hopkins University and supported by a contract from the federal government. The study determined that more than half of individuals with a diagnosis of schizophrenia who are in treatment do not receive recommended services.[1] (see p.114)

## What Do We actually Know About the Effects of Managed Care?

Managed care is one of the major forces shaping service delivery in health care generally and mental health care specifically. Managed care combines the oversight and management of individual cases with cost-containment strategies such as negotiated fees and prospective payment. It also creates networks of selected "preferred" providers who agree to the terms of practice management and financing. The utilization incentives of managed care encourage standardized services according to guidelines and protocols and the financing incentives are designed to encourage cost-effective care. Unfortunately the same incentives often just encourage less care, particularly for those with the greatest needs or the most complex conditions. In theory the incentives promote efficiency by using cost-effective, evidence-based practices. This worthy objective depends, however, on having good information to guide practice, using it faithfully, and supplying a workforce trained to deliver the evidence-based services and recognize when to use them appropriately.

Data on the experience with managed care is very incomplete. The focus is predominantly on changes in costs, demonstrating the cost reducing power of managed care incentives. Data on the impact on quality of care and outcomes is even less complete and comes only from the best implemented projects. Anecdotal evidence suggests that the routine implementation of managed care has been plagued by problems of limited access and poor quality. The general public seems increasingly to be disenchanted with managed care. A few studies raise some concern that treatment in managed care settings does not conform to evidence-based standards, but other studies suggest that the overall system's cost-effectiveness of care [at least for the acute treatment of depression] has improved over the same period as increases in care management. The improvements may be due mostly to improved technology and have occured in spite of — not because of — managed care. Whatever the impact of managed care, it is clear that the quality of care could be improved and that a workforce trained to deliver evidence-based practices is needed.

## Implementing Evidence-Based Services

There are several new initiatives to implement evidence-based practices. Some are focused on improving the treatment of depression in primary care settings, evolving from a model of chronic disease management developed at the University of Washington. This model is part of a broader approach initiated in general medicine by Edward Wagner and by his colleagues in mental health. The Robert Wood Johnson Foundation has sponsored this work both at the University of Washington and through a new program directed by Harold Pincus at the University of Pittsburgh. Other foundations have sponsored similar projects, including the MacArthur Foundation project on minor depression, based at Dartmouth [Alan Deitrich], and the Hartford Foundation projects on late life depression, based at Dartmouth and University of California at Los Angeles [Jurgen Unutzer]. The NIMH and the federal Center for Mental Health Services also have funded related projects. The largest completed project, Partners in Care, was directed by Ken Wells and Lisa Rubinstein also at UCLA. For the most part these projects are being introduced into primary care in the private sector.

There also are new public sector projects implementing evidence-based practices for individuals with severe and persistent mental disorders, such as schizophrenia. They grow out of the findings of the Schizophrenia Patient Outcome Research Team described above. One of the best documented is based at the New Hampshire-Dartmouth Psychiatric Research Center. Robert Drake directs the project, initiated with resources from the state mental health authority and a grant funded by the Robert Wood Johnson Foundation. The Evidence-Based Practices project gained more substantial funding from the federal Center for Mental Health Services and now has funding from other foundations and corporations as well. Dartmouth and New Hampshire have partnered with the NIMH-funded centers at Johns Hopkins and University of Maryland and at the National Association of State Mental Health Program Directors' Research Institute to expand the scope of the project. The activity now includes proposed demonstration sites in Maryland, Ohio, and a half dozen other states.

The Evidence-based Practices Project, described and documented throughout 2001 in *Psychiatric Services,* has three phases. The current phase involves developing "toolkits" addressing the implementation and training needs of patients, family members, clinical program managers, local mental health authorities and state mental health authorities. There are six toolkits in development, one for each of six evidence-based practices for adults with severe mental illness: medication management, family supportive psycho-education, assertive community treatment, integrated treatment for co-occurring mental and addictive disorders, supportive employment, and illness self-management. The second phase of the project proposes to study the efforts at implementing the evidence-based practices using the toolkits in the partner states - to improve the toolkits and to identify barriers and facilitators of implementation. The third phase is a proposed national demonstration with an evaluation and related research on bridging science and services.

What remains to be determined is an evidence base for quality improvement. It is essential that we develop a research foundation to guide the implementation of evidence-based practices. It is widely appreciated that there are many structural barriers to accomplishing this complex and resistant task. Regulating the incentives and creating an infrastructure to disseminate research findings, train the workforce, and implement cost-effective services is the next frontier. The concluding section of this paper examines the organizational and financing policy issues related to implementing evidence-based practices focusing special attention on the public sector as an example.

## Regulating Access to Evidence-Based Services*

*Mental Health: A Report of the Surgeon General* alerted the public, mental health advocates, and policy makers to the disparity between the opportunities for improved treatment and services and the reality of everyday practice. Scientific advances in treatment and services are not routinely available to meet the needs of individuals experiencing mental illness. The report identified "courses of action" and called on the field to "ensure the supply of mental health services and providers" and "ensure delivery of state-of-the-art treatments."

Several reports have focused attention on this public health problem and programs in the public and private sectors have offered a range of responses to the Surgeon General's call to action. Various reports and articles have documented the disparities and have reviewed individual evidence-based practices for adults and children. They have described efforts to implement them, highlighting facilitators and barriers, including rules, regulations, and mental health financing policies. This section of the paper synthesizes that material, focusing on the role of policy makers in the process of implementing evidence-based practices, particularly in the public sector.

Returning to a focus on policy brings us full circle in the process of reforming mental health services. The earliest stages of the community mental health and community support reforms emphasized organizational and financing solutions to the problems of individuals experiencing mental illness, particularly severe and persistent mental disorders. Treatment technology was comparatively weak, and the reforms focused on the locus of treatment in the community and on the system of care. Attention shifted to the content and quality of services when systems interventions alone proved necessary but insufficient to improve the lives of mentally ill individuals. Research documented both the potential benefits of services and treatments and the deficiencies in usual care. Some policies have been identified as specific barriers to implementing evidence-based services, and other policies have been identified as facilitators. Policy creates incentives and disincentives that shape the mental health service system. A major challenge is identifying policy interventions to facilitate implementation and minimize barriers to evidence-based practices. This paper is addressed to policy makers and to those who advise them and would influence their rules and regulations – namely the rest of us.

## Implementing Evidence-Based Practices to Achieve Quality and Accountability

Quality and accountability have become the watchwords of health and mental health services. Implementing evidence-based services has become a means to achieving both ends. Michael Hogan, Commissioner of Mental Health in Ohio, refers to a triangular relationship among these three service system elements: quality improvement, accountability through performance measurement, and evidence-based practices. He describes this relationship as central to providing effective mental health services. Implementing evidence-based practices is a quality improvement process providing accountability through the monitoring of the fidelity of practices to models that have been demonstrated effective by research. Using this framework, policy makers can approach their funders with greater confidence. They can argue for resources to implement evidence-practices with the assurance that funders will get "value for money" and accountability. Monitoring for adherence to evidence-based practices is possible using fidelity measures. Programs faithful to the evidence-based models produce good outcomes: that is at the heart of what is meant by an evidence-based practice. In this fashion the quality of mental health services can be continuously improved.

Unfortunately, although the Surgeon General concluded that a range of efficacious treatments exist for most every mental disorder, for many specific clinical situations there is no evidence to support treatments and services. For example, although there are effective treatments for schizophrenia and bipolar disorders, many patients with these disorders have complications and co-morbidities that have not been considered in studies of treatment effectiveness. Some problems with the greatest salience, such as youth violence or borderline personality disorder, do not yet have a satisfactory research base to guide policy and practice with clarity. Not every problem has an evidence-based solution. There continues to be much room for clinical judgment and innovative treatment and service development. Evidence-based practices, however, do exist for certain clinical circumstances. Yet, too often these practices are not implemented, even when their benefits are well understood and models exist of successful implementation.

States are moving forward in implementing evidence-based practices with varying commitment and success. Many are struggling with the implementation of evidence-based practices which have been extant for more than a decade and which have been proven to be effective in a variety of settings. Even when states have had the political and administrative will to implement evidence-based services they have not always done so with mechanisms to assure adherence to fidelity. And even when evidence-based services have been implemented with fidelity, systems must address issues as to how these fit with each other and with services that do not have a strong evidence base. It is within such a context that the policy infrastructure has paramount importance.

### Overcoming Systemic Barriers

Although the focus has shifted from organization and financing to the content and quality of services, policy makers cannot ignore the systemic barriers to implementing evidence-based practices. The literature on evidence-based practices has identified organizational and financing policy barriers to implementation, and some have identified strategies to overcome those barriers and create appropriate incentives to support implementation. We use the eight "courses of action" outlined by the Surgeon General to organize our thinking about how to implement evidence-based practices:

- ***Continue to build the science base***. As noted above, there are limitations in the treatment effectiveness research base that defines the evidence-based practices. More research is needed to determine whether these practices are effective with all ethnic sub-populations, with individuals with multiple co-morbidities, and in all practice settings [*e.g.* in rural as well as urban settings]. Furthermore, there is virtually no evidence base on how to implement evidence-based practices. There is uncomfortable irony in moving forward to implement evidence-based practice without an evidence base to guide implementation practice. Torrey reviewed some of the literature on dissemination and implementation, but there is more that we do not know than what we do know from this literature. It is better at telling us what does not work and what not to do that to guide our work. It is our intention to study the earliest experiences with the Evidence-Based Practices Project to inform future efforts at implementation.

- *Overcome stigma.* Few of the authors identified stigma as a special barrier to implementing evidence-based practices. It may be, however, that the pervasive stigma associated with mental illness and its treatment has resulted in discriminatory financing policies. All of the authors in this series have identified financing policies as barriers to implementing evidence-based practices.

- *Improve public awareness of effective treatments.* Each of the authors initiated their articles with a careful description of the evidence-based practices. It cannot be assumed that the readers of *Psychiatric Services* are all familiar with all of the evidence-based practices, themselves, let alone understand all of the barriers and facilitators of implementation. Although awareness alone is not sufficient to lead to implementation, it is certainly a necessary first step in the process. Consumers and family members can affect the demand for evidence-based practices, if they are aware of the benefits associated with their use. Providers - both clinicians and administrators - must understand the practices and their utility before they can be expected to adopt new practices. The same, of course, is true for policy makers.

- *Ensure the supply of mental health services and providers.* This and the next course of action are at the heart of the matter. Policy makers have a responsibility to ensure that individual clinicians and service providers are available within their mental health systems. This means making a commitment to recruiting individuals with the needed skills in delivering evidence-based practices, creating incentives to attract them to practice in their systems, and training, supervising and supporting the work of providers in evidence-based practices. Retaining skilled providers and minimizing job burnout are critical to maintaining a workforce capable of supplying evidence-based practices. According to the Surgeon General and the authors of this series, there is a shortage of trained personnel able to perform the evidence-based practices described. The Evidence-Based Practices Project is designed to increase the number of individuals and clinical service teams that are able to practice in a manner supported by research findings. Assertive community treatment, supported employment, integrated treatment for co-occurring substance abuse and severe mental disorder, and family supportive interventions all need skilled and well-trained professionals. The same is true for self-managed care and proper medication use. Some practices require special training for consumer providers and family members. All need informed and engaged individuals at all levels of service provision: consumers, family members, clinicians, program administrators, and policy makers.

- *Ensure delivery of state-of-the-art treatments.* Each of the authors of the papers on each of the evidence-based practices reinforced the need for leadership in implementing state-of-the-art practices. They also indicated that "ensuring delivery" is not a trivial matter. Evidence-based practices must be a priority for care. Architects of the mental health system must organize services with quality improvement in mind. Regulations often impede implementation of evidence-based practices. It is not possible to deliver state-of-the-art treatments, for example, if newer anti-psychotic medications are not in the formulary of a program or if an insurer does not cover family interventions. Regulations may create unanticipated barriers; for example, supported employment may not be an approved service for Medicaid reimbursement. Organizational barriers to integrated treatment have been identified for supported employment [between vocational rehabilitation and mental health agencies] and for integrated treatment of co-occurring substance abuse and severe mental illness [between separate substance abuse and mental health service authorities]. Overcoming these agencies divisions' is often important to beginning the effort to provide better-integrated services. On the other hand, some of these services [*e.g.* assertive community treatment] are designed to provide the services themselves rather than to rely on obtaining them from a fragmented service system.

- *Tailor treatment to age, gender, race, and culture.* Although the research base is not sufficient to support all of the evidence-based practices with each of the socio-demographic groups encountered in practice, it is always important to be culturally sensitive and respectful of diversity in service design and delivery. It is also important to realize that for the most part, when research has been conducted with ethnic sub-populations, the evidence-based practices have produced good results. The issue of tailoring treatment will be of special importance in situations where "culture counts" in specific ways. For example, family interventions must account for the cultural meanings of family and respect the differences in meaning depending on age, gender, and stage in the life cycle. Language-appropriate services are critical to successful outreach and to encourage members of linguistic minorities to use evidence-based services. Medications should be used appropriately with an awareness of ethno-psychopharmacologic variations in physiology as well as in attitudes and behaviors in relation to drug taking. In addition to being faithful to program models, evidence-based services must be inviting to everyone in a community who might need or benefit from the services.

- *Facilitate entry into treatment.* In most instances, people cannot benefit from evidence-based treatments if they do not seek help. Occasionally treatment may be provided under a court order, but in general the goal is to provide services on a voluntary basis. The evidence-based services must be available and accessible, and as noted above, they should be inviting. The Surgeon General offered the belief and hope that evidence-based practices would reduce the need for coercion in mental health services. He encouraged multiple "portals of entry" to services by creating incentives for many service providers to receive referrals and accept all individuals seeking services. Subsequently individuals can be matched with appropriate evidence-based services, provided by specially trained clinicians, teams, and programs within the service system. Not every service provider will provide all of the evidence-based services, but every clinician and provider organization should provide choices of some of the evidence-based services delivered within their organization or elsewhere in the system. There should be "no wrong door" for services. Awareness of evidence-based practices and where such services can be received is essential information for the contemporary mental health service system.

- *Reduce financial barriers to treatment.* No single policy issue received more attention from the authors of the papers on implementing evidence-based practices than the adequacy of financing. A service is not realistically available if an individual with a mental illness cannot afford to use it or a program cannot afford to provide it for the prices offered by payers. It is a simple truism that a service system runs on its financing policies. If evidence-based practices are not "covered services" or if the fees paid are below the cost of providing them, they will not be used. Until very recently Medicaid policy almost uniformly discouraged the provision of assertive community treatment; the federal block grant has made it complex to fund integrated services for individuals with co-occurring disorders. Payment for multifamily groups is not always covered or reimbursed adequately. The same may be true for various components of self-managed care. Newer medications may not be on a pharmacy benefit plan formulary or co-payments may discourage the use of newer agents. Supported employment may not be reimbursed at a favorable rate compared to a sheltered workshop. These are recurrent issues in every discussion of barriers to implementing evidence-based practices. The remedies are self-evident: remove unreasonable financial barriers. But these policies often are out of the decision-making purview of the mental health authority. Working on these policies with other agencies has become standard practice for supporting evidence-based practice implementation.

A special financing policy need is for resources to support the transition to evidence-based practices in agencies historically involved in older practices. It is difficult to be motivated to learn a new practice if the old practice generated the revenues for the agency. Funds are needed to offset the opportunity costs associated with learning a new practice. In general the move to evidence-based practices will not be accompanied by permanent additional resources. Many successful implementations have occurred when agencies switched from an older practice, such as brokering case management or rehabilitation-oriented day treatment, to assertive community treatment or supported employment. They benefit from additional one-time-only resources to support the "hump" or "model changeover" transitioning to evidence-based practices.

Cutting across all of these courses of action is the need for leadership from mental health policy makers. Most authors indicated the need for a dedicated individual and for an infrastructure to support the implementation of evidence-based practices.

## An Infrastructure to Support Systemic Change

Without evidence to guide them, various mental health authorities have developed similar infrastructure to support systemic change toward evidence-based practice and quality improvement. The Evidence-Based Practices project began in New Hampshire, Maryland and Ohio and has spread to several other States. The original three states each developed their own centers for implementing evidence-based practices, taking advantage of local opportunities and preferences. Each of the states is somewhat different and has created its own model. The Project has stimulated some cross-fertilization, so the centers share many of the same functions, but the differences are illustrative and might encourage other states to develop similar centers of their own. Each of them is sponsored at least in part by the state mental health authority. Each views its mission as supporting the implementation of evidence-based practices, involving training, supervision, ongoing clinical and administrative support in the new practice, and structural support [with regulations and financing technical assistance]. Each center sponsors needs assessment activities, training events, and various supportive services to the process of implementing evidence-based practices. The centers work with all of the related stakeholders: the state and local mental health authorities, program administrators, clinicians and other providers, consumers and their families.

In New Hampshire, the West Center for Implementing Evidence-Based Practices is a partnership between the state and a private family foundation. It grew out of the well-established public-academic linkage between the state mental health authority and Dartmouth Medical School. It is affiliated with the New Hampshire-Dartmouth Psychiatric Research Center (NH-D PRC), where several of the evidence-based practices were developed and evaluated. The Evidence-Based Practices Project is run out of the West Center and the NH-D PRC. The centralized model in New Hampshire is well suited to a small state with a single academic center.

In Maryland, the Center for Implementing Evidence-Based Practices is a newly established center within the Maryland Mental Health Service Improvement Collaborative. Sponsored by the state mental health authority, the center is an outgrowth of the original collaborative devoted to providing training and conference opportunities for service providers in Maryland. Like the New Hampshire center it is a key element of one of the oldest public-academic liaisons in the country, between the Department of Psychiatry at the University of Maryland and the Mental Hygiene Administration. The specific link is with the Center for Mental Health Services Research, which together with colleagues at the Johns Hopkins University have an National Institutes of Mental Health-funded research center that conducted the Schizophrenia Patient Outcome Research Team. The Patient Outcome Research Team study was one of the first to identify and explore the major problem with the disparity between research and practice. No private funds have yet been obtained to support the Center but a network grant from the MacArthur Foundation to the university may fund pilot research on implementing evidence-based practices in these centers.

In contrast to the centralized model employed by New Hampshire and Maryland, [both comparatively small states], Ohio uses a decentralized approach. The Coordinating Centers of Excellence are a series of centers [currently eight - ten are planned] decentralized throughout Ohio. Each is linked to a research-oriented institution - either a university or a private sector entity - specializing in one area of evidence-based practice. In Ohio, where there are multiple small research centers and where local mental health authorities are extremely important to mental health services, the decentralized and specialized approach makes the most sense. Some of Ohio's Coordinating Centers of Excellence focus on practices with substantial research evidence; others are focused on areas of policy salience [*e.g.* school-based mental health services] that cannot wait for an evidence-base to accumulate before providing some guidance to local mental health authorities.

In Texas, statewide implementation of evidence-based services has occurred through collaboration with academic centers and stakeholder groups to advocate for resources for evidence-based services and through contractual requirements (including financial sanctions) with local mental health authorities to provide evidence-based services. These collaborations have also resulted in major research initiatives related to the implementation of evidence-based services.

The National Association of State Mental Health Program Directors [NASMHPD] and the NASMHPD Research Institute, using a grant from the NIMH to advance its research work on evidence-based practice, are coordinating these efforts at the level of the state mental health authority. The NASMHPD Research Institute has created a Center on Evidence-Based Practices, Performance Measurement and Quality Improvement to support state efforts to implement evidence-based services and to monitor the quality and impact of services being provided. The functions of the center are to identify, share and promote knowledge in these areas; conduct research and develop knowledge; provide technical assistance, and coordinate activities across organizational entities and levels of government. Several additional states are involved in the Project and have their own approaches to infrastructure development. Private entities, such as the non-profit Institute of the Technical Assistance Collaborative, are emerging to provide technical assistance on infrastructure and on policies to support evidence-based practices.

## Conclusion

The time has come to add to the body of knowledge about implementing evidence-based practices at different levels including policy, program priorities, clinician practice, consumer adherence and family member support. The policy level, however, is both primary and paramount. The national initiative embodied by the Project is one of the most important innovations on the mental health horizon. It will serve as the testing ground for what one can learn about bridging science and service.

This important initiative will not go far if it is not supported by mental health policies that create the organizational and financial incentives to implement evidence-based practices. The promise of decades of research must be realized in practice. The Surgeon General simultaneously has identified the promise and documented our shortcomings. His report outlines courses of action for policy makers to guide us away from service disparities and to support implementing evidence-based practices. We have the opportunity to combine quality improvement with accountability through performance measurement and the implementation of effective new services and treatments.

One of the most important challenges remaining is to educate professionals to meet new needs as the evidence base for practice expands. The challenge goes well beyond the training of a new work force in sufficient numbers. It requires training new professionals to use effective treatments and re-training current professionals as well. There are many structural barriers to supplying the needed work-force that go well beyond education and training. Incentives to provide evidence-based care are essential to reduce the global burden of disease imposed by mental illness and to improve the mental health of the world's population.

* Substantial portions of this presentation are taken from Goldman HH *et al*: "Policy implications for implementing evidence-based practices." *Psychiatric Services* 52:1591-1597, 2001 and are used with the permission of the American Psychiatric Association.

# Integrating Neuroscience, Behavioral Science, and Genetics in Modern Psychiatry

**Steven E. Hyman, M.D.**
**Provost, Harvard University**
**(Director, National Institute of Mental Health, at the time of this presentation)**

**Abstract:** The scientific basis of psychiatry has moved beyond approaches, dating from the mid-20th century, which attempted to explain mental illness largely through single lenses, whether psychological or pharmacological. Psychodynamics, the dominant psychological approach in mid-20th century psychiatry, gave rise to a rich explanatory system strangely divorced from rigorous empirical observations or tests; early biological models based almost entirely in pharmacology were so reductionistic and impoverished as to explain little — despite empirical testing. In the last decade we have witnessed the glimmerings of a far more successful scientific approach to mental illness, the product of contributions from many disciplines, including genetics, molecular and cellular neuroscience, systems-level and cognitive neuroscience and other areas of behavioral and social science. We must not err again by underestimating the difficulties of understanding mental illnesses, disorders of the highest integrated functioning of the human brain. For example, we must be realistic about the time that will be required to identify genes that increase susceptibility to mental illness, to ascertain what those genes do within neurons, to determine what the relevant neurons do in the brain, and only then to understand how inheriting a particular version of a gene affects the risk of a mental disorder. It will be similarly challenging to determine how a life experience affects neural circuits and the neurons within them to activate molecular processes of plasticity that will, in turn, alter cognition or behavior. These and other challenges notwithstanding, there are increasingly well marked scientific paths that ultimately will help us to better understand, treat, and even prevent mental illness. These prospects for the science of mental illness pose critical questions for the discipline of psychiatry. Will psychiatry facilitate the application of modern scientific approaches to mental illness by its embrace of stronger models of brain and behavior and by efforts to assure a rich cross-pollination of preclinical science with clinical investigation? Or, at the other extreme, will the profession slow progress by clinging to increasingly frayed models of psychopathology and by discouraging the production of skilled investigators? In this latter scenario — much to be avoided — our patients will ultimately suffer while psychiatry spends additional decades standing on the sidelines of mainstream biomedical and behavioral research.

## Introduction

After decades of frustration in which psychiatry lacked the tools necessary to understand the pathogenesis of mental disorders or to develop treatments based on knowledge rather than the enlightened exploitation of serendipity, we now find ourselves at the dawn of a new scientific era. This dawn is not likely to prove illusory because it is not based on inflated hopes that some single new approach will provide a magical key to understanding broad swaths of psychopathology. In contrast to the recent past, ranging from the era of psychoanalysis to that of early biological psychiatry (which, in fact, ignored most of the richness of biology and behavioral science), the field today soberly recognizes the complexity of the brain and behavior. For example, mainstream biology has recognized the importance of the genome to the risk of mental disorders and to the promise of developing new treatments, but at the same time recognizes the enormous complexity of genetics and anticipates the challenges of mining the genome for knowledge. The current hopes for progress in psychiatry are not based on a single scientific approach, but are grounded in the real and steady progress that has been made across many disciplines in biology and behavioral science. Diverse tools being developed throughout the scientific enterprise are likely to prove relevant to psychiatric research; the question before us today is whether our discipline will harness them effectively and in a timely way in the service of people with mental illness.

In this brief presentation, it would be neither feasible nor useful to list every significant technological and methodological advance of promise to our field. Instead, I will highlight a few of the major new developments that are having important impacts on research in psychiatry; these developments can illustrate both the promise and the difficulties of the relevant science and highlight the challenges for psychiatry.

## Genetics

Identifying genetic risk factors for illnesses such as schizophrenia, autism, and bipolar disorder is imperative because genes, in aggregate, are responsible for a large proportion of the risk for each of these conditions. This means that gene identification will provide to psychiatry, as to all of medicine, critically important scientific tools for understanding pathogenesis and for developing new treatments (Subramanian *et al.*, 2001) as is already well under way for simple "Mendelian" disorders of the nervous system, *i.e.* disorders caused by a single gene (Cummings and Zoghbi, 2000). There now exist excellent working drafts of the human genome sequence as well as the sequences of many vitally important model organisms (Lander *et al.*, 2001; Venter *et al.*, 2001). However, the identification of versions of genes (alleles) that increase risk of mental illness requires more than a reference human sequence. Since genetics is based on correlating genetic variation with phenotypic variation, we also need an exhaustive catalog of human genetic variation. The sequencing of many human chromosomal regions has yielded an informative catalogue of human genetic diversity in the form of single base changes in DNA, which turn out to be the most common type of variation in the genome. These are most commonly described as single nucleotide polymorphisms, or SNPs (Sachidanandam *et al.*, 2001).

Methods that will permit us to put this catalogue of SNPs to work effectively are emerging more rapidly than could have been anticipated a few years ago. For example, it is becoming evident that in different human populations, blocks of DNA (called haplotypes) are inherited whole, reflecting the youth of the human species and the fact that chromosomal recombination at meiosis appears to occur predominantly at certain "hot spots" (Daly *et al.*, 2001; Patil *et al.*, 2001). Each of these haplotypes can be defined and marked with a small number of SNPs. With the development of improved statistical models and cheaper, more rapid methods of DNA sequencing, it should be possible to perform powerful whole genome association studies which seek to correlate combinations of haplotypes with human phenotypes, including mental disorders. With such information, the path to identifying the critical gene or genes that affect susceptibility to mental illness within identified DNA regions is becoming increasingly straightforward, Despite this increasingly powerful technology, I am not suggesting that in short order we will proceed to identify the genetic variants that produce risk of mental illnesses. In fact, the genetics of mental disorders turns out to be fiendishly complex. Current models suggest that, for each mental disorder that has been well studied (*e.g.*, schizophrenia, autism, or bipolar disorder), multiple genetic variants and nongenetic factors must interact — likely in non-additive fashion — to produce illness. For example, Risch *et al.* (1999) have suggested that at least 10 distinct genetic loci may play a role in susceptibility to autism. Moreover, there likely are heterogeneous paths to similar phenotypes; that is, no single genetic variant may be either necessary or sufficient to produce illness. Of course, behavioral scientists, neuroscientists, and clinicians must also hold up their end of the bargain by helping geneticists to get a better handle on mental illness phenotypes, an issue which has proved far from simple. Genes play a critical role not only in the risk of mental illness but also in normal brain development (Thompson *et al.*, 2001a) and therefore, normal behavioral variation including such phenotypes as temperaments which are also extremely challenging to define. Despite the difficulties with both genotypes and phenotypes, there are sensible and productive ways of proceeding, and ultimately, we are likely to succeed in identifying highly informative risk genes. It should be noted that the difficulties facing psychiatry are not unique. All of medicine faces similar complexities in understanding the genetic susceptibility factors for such common diseases such as asthma, diabetes, hypertension, or coronary artery disease. The disadvantage for psychiatry — and not a trivial one — is the lack of objective diagnostic tests to anchor important phenotypes. The bottom line for psychiatry, however, is that for the first time technologies exist that will permit psychiatric gene hunters to succeed. Those technologies do not make success automatic, however, and will require concerted efforts to bring together multiple scientific disciplines.

The sequencing of the genome is simply the best-known aspect of a fundamental new frontier in biology. With the identification of all DNA sequences, there are new efforts to identify all of the messenger RNAs (mRNAs) that the genome encodes, and to develop collections representing the full complement of RNAs produced by the cells of the human body, and of other organisms across the lifetime. This exhaustive catalog of RNAs representing the "transcriptome", and similar attempts to identify the full complement of proteins within the "proteome" are being combined with powerful new tools to create new systematic approaches to biology. Until now, biologists studied one gene, RNA, or protein at a time. This new biology makes it possible to study global patterns of gene expression (functional genomics) or patterns of protein expression (proteomics). One important approach to functional genomics is based on use of DNA microarrays ("chips" spotted with thousands of complementary DNA copies of transcribed RNAs and ultimately with a representation of the entire transcriptome) to study global changes in gene expression. Microarrays are already in wide use in fundamental neuroscience to study development, neurotransmitter or drug responses, and disease processes. In psychiatry, post-mortem human brain tissue is being studied with DNA microarrays, *e.g.*, to make comparisons of global patterns of gene expression in brains from individuals with schizophrenia versus controls (Mirnics *et al.*, 2000). These technologies also are being used to study psychotropic drug responses in animal models, at the level of altered gene expression. The major stumbling blocks for psychiatry are not likely to lie in the genomic technologies, which are developing rapidly, but rather in the characterization of the patient samples and in the thoughtful analysis of the enormous amounts of data that will be produced. Genetics and functional genomics are spurring rapid development of what is being called computational biology so that data can be mined for significant information. In the next few years functional genomics and the nascent field of proteomics will complement older tools in helping us to understand brain development, brain function, brain plasticity, and brain disease.

Another important development based in genetics and molecular biology is the already powerful ability to insert and delete genes from the mouse genome. Increasingly, it has been possible to control where and when in the brain a particular gene and its protein product will be expressed. Although few believe that there can be ideal mouse models of depression or schizophrenia, there may be partial models of great utility. Already, for example, very useful mouse models have been produced for Alzheimer disease (Price *et al.*, 2000) and Rett syndrome (Guy, *et al.*, 2001), a rare Mendelian disorder that has features of autism. These models were produced by the insertion of human mutations discovered by human genetics into the mouse genome. Such models will be critical tools for developing hypotheses about pathogenesis, and also for the development of new treatments and preventive interventions. Other genetic approaches to mouse models and other animal models are well underway. Because for psychiatry the critical phenotypes of mouse mutants involve behavior, it is urgent to address shortages of scientists with great sophistication about animal behavior and its relation to brain function.

## Gene-environment interactions

As should be clear, genes are fundamental and an understanding of genes is critical to the science of psychiatry, but it is important to recall that it is not genes per se, but the nervous system that controls mental life and behavior. The neural circuits of the brain are not only activated by experience, they are physically altered by experience, by physiological processes, by pharmacologic agents, and by illness. Experience-dependent physical change in the nervous system underlies the processes of learning and memory (Kandel, 2001) that, along with genetic diversity, underlies our individuality, a good measure of psychopathology— and the effectiveness of psychotherapy.

Understanding how this lifetime of gene-environment interactions shapes mental life and behavior is an important goal for psychiatry. This will require that we not only understand the actions of genes, but also the biology of cells, synapses, and circuits. At the same time, we must understand brain and behavior from the "top down", for example, the action of context and experience on modifying neural circuits, synapses, cells, and gene expression. We must learn how changes occur at each of these levels during normal brain development and how such processes are modified by experience and by illness. For psychiatry this will require a commitment to biology and behavioral science that employs reductionist strategies when tactically necessary, but which does not ultimately have reductionist goals. Moreover, it is important that the science of psychiatry does not isolate itself from the rest of science just as the genomic revolution is bringing all of the life sciences closer together.

**Systems Level and Cognitive Neuroscience**

Complementing the "bottom-up" molecular and cellular approaches broadly outlined above are "top down approaches" to brain and behavior. Tools to investigate the underpinnings of behavior at the neural systems level include non-invasive neuroimaging tools in both humans and, of great importance, in animal models, including primates (Logothetis, *et al.*, 1999), where they can be combined with invasive single unit recordings and multi-electrode arrays. Magnetic resonance imaging (MRI) is rapidly affording clearer views of both brain structure and function. At the level of brain structure, MRI is being used to produce atlases that depict normal brain structure across development stages and alterations in brain structure produced by disease. Computational tools for parcellation of brain regions and tools for comparisons across individuals and within a single individual over time are becoming increasingly sophisticated. It now is possible, for example, to document the progression of abnormalities in the cerebral cortical gray matter in individuals with childhood onset schizophrenia (Thompson *et al.*, 2001b). Such structural neuroimaging, which involves the collaboration of clinicians, imagers, computational biologists, and neuroanatomists, is being complemented by functional neuroimaging, a field that requires the collaboration with another critically important field, cognitive neuroscience.

Cognitive science developed as an approach to understanding the processing of information in the brain. With the recognition that models of information processing markedly increased in value when coupled to investigation of underlying brain circuitry, cognitive neuroscience was born. To understand cognitive, emotional, and behavioral disorders it matters that we learn precisely how the brain performs relevant functions, and how its processing strategy is altered by both illness and treatment. Of great importance to psychiatry, in more recent years, cognitive neuroscience has expanded its purview beyond such traditionally "cognitive" topics as sensory processing, speech, and memory to emotion (Vuilleumier *et al*, 2001), and even to aspects of interpersonal interaction (Frith 2001). Indeed a new term "social neuroscience" is being used to describe the study of how the brain underlies and is modified by interactions among persons. The combination of cognitive neuroscience and neuroimaging, together with invasive electrophysiological studies in primates is already giving us a new view of system-level neurobiology. The large "functional" brain regions of traditional neuropsychology, born of studying brain lesions, are being analyzed into far smaller modules that are connected with each other to form the distributed circuits that are most proximate to behavior. Experimental designs derived from cognitive neuroscience are now frequently coupled with neuroimaging in clinical populations to attempt to identify particular aspects of mental function and its neural underpinnings that reflect specific disorders. Similar approaches are being undertaken to help explicate neural responses to treatment. It is very early in such investigations, but the sophisticated use of systems-level neuroscience, cognitive neuroscience, and imaging can make a powerful contribution to the science of psychiatry.

## Epidemiology, Diagnosis, and Clinical Investigations

The proliferation of new ideas is not limited to the more basic areas of psychiatric science. New information emerging from genetics and the study of other risk factors demands changes in psychiatry's approaches to diagnosis, epidemiology, and even clinical trials. With respect to the latter, it is no longer possible to perform a relatively small trial on a narrowly-defined population recruited at an academic health center for limited period of time (typically eight to ten weeks) and, on that basis, conclude that a treatment "works". Questions about the generalizability of treatments, both pharmacologic and psychosocial, require the design of subsequent trials that will involve the more heterogeneous populations likely to be encountered in actual clinical practice settings, including the primary care sector. There is growing awareness, too, that treatment outcome must be assessed over a considerably longer timeframe than was accepted in the past and that functional outcomes must supplement measure of symptom reduction. Of course, with each new variable the statistical power of clinical trials is progressively eroded. Thus, psychiatry needs clinical investigators to look anew at the methodologies that were considered to have reached their apex decades ago with development of the randomized, double-blind, placebo-controlled clinical trial.

## Implications of the Evolving Science Base for Psychiatry Education

The need for the ability to wield the tools of genetics, computational biology, molecular, cellular, systems level, and cognitive neuroscience, epidemiology, clinical trials design and other fields, and to translate them into the arena of clinical psychiatric research has never been more pressing for a single reason: never have the opportunities to benefit patients with mental disorders been greater. Optimism about the burgeoning tools of science and fundamentally new ideas, which match tools and technologies in their power, is tempered, however, by legitimate concern about the capacity of psychiatry to use the advances appropriately and effectively. There are two areas of concern. The first is that at the level of practice. To date, modern genetics, neuroscience, and behavioral science have little impact on the thinking or practice of most front-line clinical psychiatrists. Information about genetics and neurobiology that is presented in most training programs is too often outdated, or, if up-to-date, so arcane as to seem irrelevant to clinical practice. In fact, the model that a psychiatrist holds of how a person's illness came to be matters greatly. Cartesian caricatures have not yet been fully banished: for example, the idea that there are disorders primarily of psychosocial origin that should be treated with psychosocial therapies: and disorders primarily of biological origin that should receive pharmacotherapy or other somatic treatments. Far too many psychiatrists hold outdated understandings of the roles of genes and the functions of the brain; all too few are familiar with the relevant literature of modern cognitive science and social psychology. This knowledge gap has implications not only for treatment, but may negatively affect the ability of psychiatry to attract the brightest medical students to enter the profession, whether as clinicians or as scientists.

A second problem confronting psychiatry concerns the training of psychiatrists who might undertake independent research careers. Because the neuroscience and genetics of thought, of emotion, and behavior are intrinsically interesting and possess enviable tools and ideas, these areas of science certainly will continue to make progress. A real possibility exists, however, that accumulating knowledge about basic processes will not be rapidly or effectively translated into clinical applications, unless our profession can improve its ability to recruit and effectively train young investigators.

Certain of the obstacles to communicating sophisticated new scientific knowledge to psychiatric trainees and practitioners are based on a problem that exists across the entire breadth of medicine. With progress, much of science has grown farther from clinical practice and its language more technical and forbidding. Textbook knowledge has become quantitatively overwhelming and in psychiatry its direct relevance to patients and their treatment still is rather indirect. Better textbooks are part of the solution, but the real answer lies in different approaches to teaching science to medical students and residents as well as practicing clinicians. The new approaches must not be segregated into isolated nooks and crannies of the curriculum or occasional seminars or grand rounds, but must be an integral part of the broad platform of medical education and psychiatry specialty training. This is a difficult set of problems that will require the field to develop living and relevant curricular materials that are better related to the clinical situation and to provide better training opportunities for teaching faculty.

How might psychiatry more effectively attract future researchers to its ranks? According to the American Psychiatric Association, the number of U.S. medical graduates matching to psychiatry over the past decade has dropped from 641 in 1991 to 524 in 2001. Of these, less than ten percent express interest in academic or research careers upon entering training and, ultimately, only a small fraction of these will pursue the rigors of an independent scientific career. The arithmetic is tragically straightforward: The number of psychiatrists who will be successfully engaged in science in the coming decades is approaching zero, this despite the incredible opportunities that have been briefly sketched above. Of course, U.S. medical graduates are not the only source for psychiatric science, but the issue of recruiting the brightest foreign medical graduates to careers in psychiatric science is an area in which we have even less control.

Psychiatry begins at a disadvantage with respect to other areas of medicine in terms of its exposure in the undergraduate medical curriculum. This results from the recency of the emergence of our science, from the historical stigmatization and marginalization of mental disorders, and from the recent history of psychoanalytic dominance, which made psychiatry appear extremely different from other medical specialties. While we should be aided by our maturing science and by the staggering public health burden created by mental disorders, history is difficult to overcome in a packed curriculum. I would argue that one very important goal for our field is to ensure that those individuals who are selected by psychiatry departments to instruct medical students, either in the preclinical or clinical portions of the curriculum, be outstanding teachers who are well-supported by their departments, and who have an opportunity to be steeped in modern psychiatric science. This is not a suggestion that psychiatry eschew the important aspects of understanding and teaching the physician-patient relationship or diminish the intrinsic humanism of this profession. However, failure to select and support scientifically strong instructors will imperil the ability of the profession to attract strong trainees, among them those who will be most important in the scientific progress of the field. Departments with research programs also should aggressively pursue the recruitment of outstanding medical students and foster their appreciation for the intellectual challenges and excitement of psychiatry's research questions. It is a truism that good mentoring will often go a long way toward creating a life-long interest in a problem or a discipline.

If the goal is to participate fully in mainstream biomedical and behavioral research and its translation to the problems of mental illness, it is critical that we not only attract bright students into psychiatric residency, but that residency training offers an entrée into modern science. Psychiatry residents should have the opportunity to be exposed to cutting edge genetics, neuroscience, behavioral science, epidemiology, and clinical trials design—both so that they can have a sense of mastery over the literature and also to attract a subset into research. As a field we should ensure that appropriate research experiences are available to residents and fellows, including the possibility of training outside of the psychiatry department if necessary. It is difficult for any medical school department to maintain a faculty fully capable of instructing students in the diverse areas critical to modern medicine; thus, departments of medicine and, to a substantial degree, departments of neurology long have had the tradition of permitting promising fellows to train in a science outside of the clinical department and then creating a "start up package" to encourage the return of these young people as physician-investigators. This, unfortunately is not a tradition in most psychiatry departments. Concern that once residents leave the department they might be lost to psychiatry is ultimately self-defeating insofar as it plays out in our inability to generate an adequate supply of investigators who can translate modern genetics, neuroscience, or cognitive neuroscience into clinical research on mental illness. The field needs to take the long view, which is that we should do everything in our power to help incorporate the best of modern science into our discipline. As a result of retaining too many of our small number of research trainees within psychiatry departments we have, perhaps, a surfeit of trainees focused on older areas of pharmacology and too few focused on statistical genetics, systems level neuroscience, cognitive neuroscience, or at the cutting edge of clinical trials design, to name a few very important areas.

## Conclusion

Psychiatry has entered an era of enormous opportunity but has stepped over the threshold without having made an adequate attempt to think through its place in medical school curricula or to reform residency training. Lacking that effort, many extraordinary opportunities will slip away to the detriment of our patients. We need to do a better job of attracting talented people into strengthened residencies that provide not only essential skills in the doctor-patient relationship but also in evidence-based practice, and with a strong grounding in science. We also need to devise innovative ways to encourage a subset of talented residents to go on to effective, independent research careers. We have to think about ways in which we can provide a stronger intellectual environment and support for training programs, not only for research-oriented residents but for all residents; and then we have to work as a community to permit a seamless transition to research training and a research career for those who want it.

## References:


Cummings, C.J., Zoghbi, H.Y. (2000) Trinucleotide repeats: Mechanisms and Pathophysiology. *Annual Review of Genomics and Human Genetetics*, 1: 281-328.

Daly, M.J., Rioux, J.D., Schaffner, S.F., Hudson, T.J., Lander, E.S. (2001) High-resolution haplotype structure in the human genome. *Nat Genet*, 29: 229-32.

Frith, U. Mind blindness and the brain in autism. (2001) *Neuron*, 32: 969-979.

Guy, J., Hendrich, B., Holmes, M., Martin, J.E., and Bird, A. (2001) A mouse Mecp2-null mutation causes neurological symptoms that mimic Rett syndrome. *Nature Genet*, 27: 322-326.

Kandel E.R. (2001) The molecular biology of memory storage: a dialogue between genes and synapses *Science*, 294:1030-8.

Lander, E.S., *et al.* (2001) Initial sequencing and analysis of the human genome. *Nature*, 409: 860-921.

Logothetis, N.K., Guggenberger, H., Peled S., Pauls J. (1999) Functional imaging of the monkey brain. *Nat Neurosci*, 2: 555-562

Mirnics, K., Middleton, F.A., Marquez, A., Lewis, D.A., and Levitt, P. (2000) Molecular characterization of schizophrenia viewed by microarray analysis of gene expression in prefrontal cortex. *Neuron*, 28: 53-67.

Patil, N., Berno, A.J., Hinds, D.A., Barrett, W.A., Doshi, J.M., Hacker, C.R., Kautzer, C.R., Lee, D.H., Marjoribanks, C., McDonough, D.P., Nguyen, B.T., Norris, M.C., Sheehan, J.B., Shen, N., Stern, D., Stokowski, R.P., Thomas, D.J., Trulson, M.O., Vyas, K.R., Frazer, K.A., Fodor, S.P., Cox, D.R. (2001) Blocks of limited haplotype diversity revealed by high-resolution scanning of human chromosome 21. *Science*, 294: 1719-1723.

Price, D.L., Wong, P.C., Markowska, A.L., Lee, M.K., Thinakaren, G., Cleveland, D.W., Sisodia, S.S., Borchelt, D.R. (2000) The value of transgenic models for the study of neurodegenerative diseases. *Ann N Y Acad Sci.* 920: 179-91.

Risch, N., Spiker, D., Lotspeich, L., *et al.* (1999) A genomic screen of autism: evidence for a multilocus etiology. *Am J Hum Genet*, 65: 493-507.

Sachidanandam, R., *et al.* (2001) A map of human genome sequence variation containing 1.42 million single nucleotide polymorphisms. *Nature*, 409: 928-33.

Subramanian, G., Adams, M.D., Venter, J.C., Broder, S. (2001) Implications of the human genome for understanding human biology and medicine. *JAMA*, 286: 2296-2307.

Thompson, P.M., Cannon, T.D., Narr, K.L., van Erp, T., Poutanen, V.P., Huttunen, M., Lonnqvist, J., Standertskjold-Nordenstam, C.G., Kaprio, J., Khaledy, M., Dail, R., Zoumalan, C.I., Toga, A.W. (2001) Genetic influences on brain structure. *Nat Neurosci*, 4: 1253-58.

Thompson, P.M., Vidal, C., Giedd, J.N., *et al* (2001) Mapping adolescent brain change reveals dynamic wave of accelerated gray matter loss in very early-onset schizophrenia. *Proc Natl Acad Scie* (USA), 98: 11650-11655.

Venter, J.C., *et al.* (2001) The sequence of the human genome. *Science*, 291: 1304-51.

Vuilleumier, P., Armony, J.L., Driver, J., Dolan, R.J. (2001) Effects of attention and emotion on face processing in the human brain: an event-related fMRI study. *Neuron*, 30: 829-41.

## Discussion Highlights, Session I

### Recruitment & Development of Mental Health Personnel

— To meet future needs, those in the field must think about recruitment and how to redeploy the workforce. Perhaps potential professionals can be recruited at an earlier age. Experience with children and computers shows that vast amounts of highly technical information that can be absorbed at a young age. The same may be true of neuroscience if academic training regressed one step into college. There's no reason that college students cannot come into medical school already prepared with basic neuroscience information.

### Training

— Attention needs to be given to mentoring, who does it and how it is done, and the perceived threats to front line workers, many of whom have no graduate degrees. Authoritarianism and anti-intellectualism must be avoided as information is taught and disseminated to those who actually work with patients.

### Academic Health Centers (Research Funding)

— Yet there is optimism about enhancing the science base, with new evidence-based classifications of mental disorders that take into account the life course of an illness, genetic complexity, disability and chronicity, and seek to answer such questions as whether depression in a child is the same as in an elderly person or how the expression of illness is shaped by neuroplasticity. Funding for this kind of research is robust but findings must be translated into advances for patients. Bridging that gap is a political process—something neither researchers nor clinicians do well. The case needs to be made to a wide audience that mental disorders are real, that they are treatable, and that they are treatable with finite resources. To make that case politically, both efficacy and cost effectiveness must be demonstrated.

### Academic Health Centers

— The long term survival of mental health as a field depends on the survival of academic health centers whose resources shape the field and support the next generation. The survival of these centers is not a foregone conclusion.

## Health Economics

— Financial disincentives and the length of training has diminished the number of physicians interested in neurosciences and genetics at a time when it is increasingly necessary to bridge the growing gap between science and clinical practice. No field of medicine has successfully bridged that gap and no strategies have been developed to bring together researchers and clinicians in a way that is not patronizing to clinicians. C.P. Snow talked about the two-world problems with science and the humanities, but today there is a growing two-world gap between front line clinicians and the scientific underpinnings of psychiatry.

— Debunking the myth that any single gene could be etiological in a specific condition is a mark of progress and greater understanding of multiple genes and their interaction with environment should lead to better diagnostic approaches. But an educational crisis looms, for clinicians, students and practitioners fail to understand the power of the new genomics. Educational reform, starting with the basic genetic, epidemiological and ethical building blocks, is needed to provide a framework for understanding the power of the new genomics.

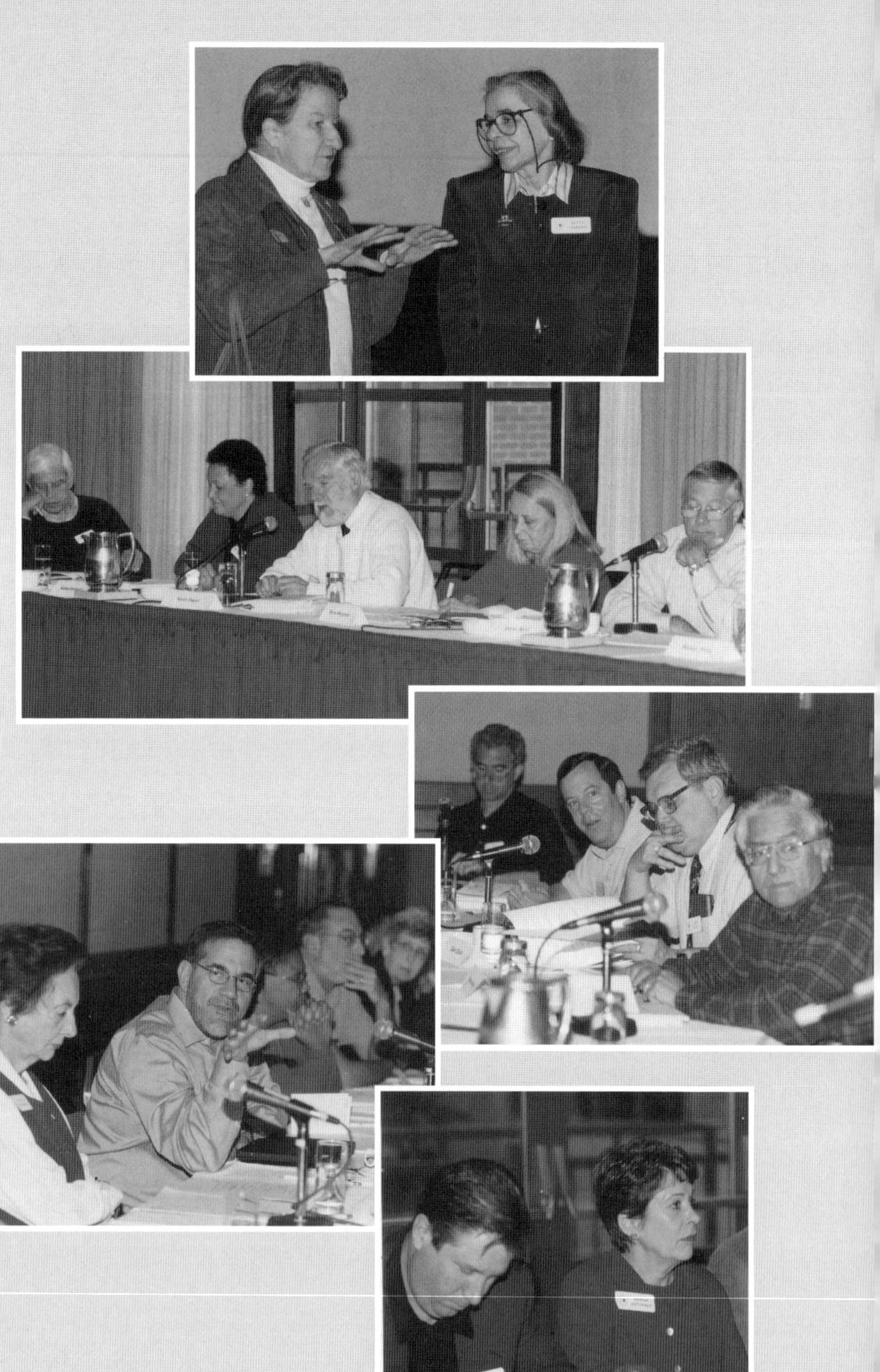

# Session II

## Bridging Research, Education and Practice

*This session highlighted significant lags in the adoption of major advances in therapeutic modalities beyond or in concert with psychopharmacology. First, the evidence-based, manualized cognitive psychotherapies were discussed, including their use by non-medical mental health professionals. Second, the critical importance of adoption of new models for comprehensive, integrated care of patients using a team approach was presented with examples of patients with dual diagnosis. Third, new approaches to the social and the community treatment of the large population of deinstitutionalized mentally ill was considered.*

# Promises and Problems in Modern Psychotherapy: the Need for Increased Training in Evidence-Based Treatments

**Myrna M. Weissman, Ph.D.**
**Professor of Epidemiology in Psychiatry,**
**Chief Division of Clinical and Genetic Epidemiology,**
**College of Physicians and Surgeons of Columbia University and The New York State Psychiatric Institute**

**William C. Sanderson, Ph.D.**
**Associate Professor of Psychology, Rutgers University**
**Department of Psychology – Graduate School of Applied and Professional Psychology**

## Abstract

Over the last 15 years there has been considerable progress in the specification of psychotherapy and then testing it in controlled clinical trials. As a result, there is an increased availability of evidence-based psychotherapy (EBT) and an increased recommendation for its use in official treatment guidelines. Data from the Medical Expenditure Panel Survey (see Appendix) shows that the demand for psychotherapy has not lessened over the last decade. However, the number of visits has decreased, psychotherapy is more often used in combination with medication, and there has been an increase in the number of patients seeing non-medically trained therapists, especially social workers. There is a clear gap between these research developments, practice guidelines, and the actual training in EBT for the three major providers (psychiatrists, psychologists and social workers). If research advances in the practice of psychotherapy are to be translated into improving services on a large scale, an accelerated change in the education and training of practitioners is needed. This paper will review the advances in specifying the essential ingredients of psychotherapy, training therapists for research studies, and the efficacy of these treatments from controlled clinical trials. To the limited extent that this information is available, the content of psychotherapy training programs (*i.e.*, residency, graduate school) and continuing education requirements will be examined to determine the level of training in EBTs. Recommendations for closing the research and practice gaps include:

1. A systematic review of residency and graduate training programs in psychiatry, psychology and social work, with an emphasis on determining the current status of training in EBT.

2. A systematic updated review of the psychotherapy efficacy and effectiveness studies with a focus on the process used to educate and train therapists.

3. Assembly of the training decision makers in psychiatry, psychology and social work to review the data from recommendations 1 and 2 with a view towards developing policy and model curriculum.

4. Assembly of the key decision makers in the three professions to review and develop continuing education criteria and policy.

5. Expansion of residency and graduate training programs to include procedures in systematic assessment and patient evaluations that are part of EBT and expansion of graduate curricula for non-medical professionals to include information on psychotropic medication and indications for referrals.

6. Specific suggestions for training therapists in evidence-based procedures.

## I. Introduction

Although we are not certain about what goes on in the real-world practice of psychotherapy, what hints we have suggest that there is a substantial discrepancy between the availability of psychotherapies with evidence for efficacy (based on controlled clinical trials) and their use in clinical practice by the three professional groups providing most of the psychotherapy: psychiatrists, psychologists and social workers (*e.g.*, Taylor, King, & Margraf, 1989; Goisman, Warshaw, & Keller, 1999; Plante, Andersen, & Boccaccini, 1999; Addis & Krasnow, 2000; Sanderson, Hiatt, & Schwartz, 2001). The discrepancy between research evidence and clinical practice begins with the education and training of practitioners. In part, this is due to the recency of the evidence base for psychotherapy. However, if research advances in the practice of psychotherapy are to be translated into improving treatment services on a large scale, an accelerated change in the education and training of practitioners is needed.

This paper will make the following points: 1) There have been significant advances in the technology and testing of psychotherapy. 2) Evidence-based psychotherapeutic treatments (EBT) exist for the range of psychiatric disorders. 3) These treatments are somewhat different than traditional psychodynamic or supportive approaches in that they are usually time-limited, specified in manuals and tested in clinical trials. 4) Psychotherapists are not using evidence-based approaches, mainly because many, perhaps the majority, of clinical graduate/residency training programs do not emphasize training in them. 5) Training programs are not emphasizing treatments endorsed by Clinical Practice Guidelines which have been developed to increase quality of care. 6) The failure to train students, the future practitioners, in EBT will leave psychotherapy vulnerable in the new health care environment, where accountability is paramount. 7) Improvement in the dissemination of evidence-based approaches needs to begin with the education of the next generation of health professionals. Current practitioners can "catch up" with guided continuing education programs. However, no criteria for the content or quality of these programs in EBT exist.

## II. Definitions and Rationale for Focus

We use the term *psychotherapy* to refer to a host of different approaches with differing theoretical and conceptual underpinnings conducted by a range of professionals with differing educational backgrounds and training. By psychotherapy, we mean an intervention in which a verbal exchange between a therapist and a patient or client is the main mode of treatment. By evidence-based treatment (EBT), we mean psychotherapy that has been defined in a manual and tested for efficacy in a controlled clinical trial. When we describe EBT we also include the systematic diagnostic and clinical monitoring assessments that are part of EBT.

While the Macy Conference entitled the program "*Modern Psychiatry*," challenges in educating health professionals was the full topic. We will follow their implicit lead and focus not only on psychiatrists but also on psychologists and social workers.

As of the year 2000, the mental health worker data indicated that there were approximately 40,000 psychiatrists, 58,000 psychologists and 155,000 social workers in the U.S. While we realize that not all of these mental health professionals practice psychotherapy, there is evidence to suggest that a large number of adults receive psychotherapy from all three. The evidence comes from a national survey (Medical Expenditure Panel Survey-MEPS) which was conducted by the Agency for Health Care Research and Quality (AHRQ). The survey was based on a national probability sample of approximately 35,000 individuals in 14,000 households (An expanded description of methods and relevant results of our analysis of the survey data can be found in the Appendix.). The survey found that 3.2% of the adult population reported receiving psychotherapy in 1987 and 3.6% reported receiving psychotherapy in 1997 (no significant difference between years). However, visiting a medical doctor (psychiatrists were not separated out in the survey in 1997) or social worker became more common; seeing a psychologist remained the same and seeing another type of non-M.D. provider became less common. Although the "popularity" of psychotherapy (as reflected by the number of persons seeing a professional for psychotherapy) did not increase from 1987 to 1997, those receiving psychotherapy in 1997 (as compared to 1987) had significantly fewer visits (see Table 1 in the Appendix). The likelihood of psychotherapy users receiving psychotropic medication nearly doubled (31% in 1987 to 58% in 1997) (see Table 2 in the Appendix). These data, to the extent they reflect current practice, suggest that short-term psychotherapy administered by non-M.D.s combined with medication is the new trend in treatment. Since psychiatrists were not separated out from medical doctors it is likely that the increase in psychotherapy sought from M.D.s reflects an increase in use of primary care physicians. The data suggest that training M.D.s and non-M.D.s in EBT is needed if the scientific advances are to be effectively translated into scientifically sound therapeutic and preventive programs.

## III. Advances in Psychotherapy

The increased availability of efficacy data on psychotherapy has largely been due to developments over the last 15 years in the specification of the essential treatment strategies in manuals and the development of programs to standardize the training of therapists providing treatment in these trials. While some practitioners in the field who received adequate training use some of these procedures, training in these procedures has not become an integral part of most educational programs (*e.g.*, graduate school, residency). As a result, in many cases, the availability of these treatments is limited to clinical research centers where the treatment is being evaluated.

Specifying Treatment in Manuals. At one time, the diversity of psychotherapists' approaches to patients discouraged research on psychotherapy. Each therapist and patient was considered unique. There was no way to define what was going on in the office with a given patient. Psychotherapy was considered an art that could not be addressed by science. Treatment manuals constitute a marked departure from this thinking and a small revolution in the ability to conduct clinical trials. Manuals operationalize the procedures in that they provide technical specifications with scripts for interventions and guidelines on what should be covered (Hibbs & Jensen, 1996; Luborsky & DuRubeis, 1984). Treatment manuals can teach experienced psychotherapists to adapt their styles to a particular approach. Audiotaping or videotaping provides an objective record of how the therapist delivers the treatment, allowing raters to review and score for treatment adherence. A manual can make psychotherapy a relatively uniform, and thus testable, treatment.

Manuals have become a virtual requirement for psychotherapy studies. Some studies have shown that the therapist's degree of adherence to the manual is significantly associated with patient improvement. In order to facilitate dissemination of EBT, a list of manuals and information on how to obtain them has been compiled (Woody & Sanderson, 1998). While over 100 EBT manuals for adult psychiatric disorders have been identified (cf. Chambless & Ollendick, 2001), a large majority of them are adaptations of cognitive behavioral therapy (CBT) and to a lesser extent, interpersonal psychotherapy (IPT). The modifications were made in order to apply the treatment to a clinical presentation of a particular disorder or age group. CBT and IPT will be described later.

**Training Therapists.** Procedures for training therapists to administer these "manualized" treatments have been developed in order to accelerate their testing in clinical trials (Shaw *et al.*, 1999; Weissman *et al.*, 2000). Typically, training programs involve: (a) the reading of the manual, (b) attendance at a didactic course, (c) supervision of several cases by a clinician trained in the approach using actual video or audio tapes of the sessions, and (d) evaluation of competence. There is evidence that reading a manual alone is not a substitute for psychotherapy training and that supervised clinical experience is critical. From a practical perspective, this is best accomplished in graduate or residency programs when therapists in training are being supervised regularly. It is possible to develop well-planned continuing education programs to fill this need for practitioners in the field. A manual does not teach therapists basic psychotherapy skills such as how to listen, hear, empathize, and handle one's own feelings and distortions. Manuals teach trained therapists a particular strategy. It is relatively easy for experienced therapists to learn specified therapies. The limitations are usually only ideologic.

**Evaluating Treatments.** Treatment manuals, training programs, and therapist competency criteria maximized internal validity and were necessary technologies to begin testing the efficacy of psychotherapy in controlled clinical trials. As a result of these efforts, there has been a substantial increase during the past 15 years in the number and quality of studies supporting the efficacy of several psychotherapies. These EBTs cover the full range of psychiatric disorders. Efficacy studies evaluating treatment manuals is an essential link in determining how well a treatment works for a given disorder (cf. Chambless *et al.*, 1998; Nathan & Gorman, 1998; Weissman *et al.*, 2000).

The next challenge is to determine how well these treatments generalize to clinical practice where patients often do not have a single diagnosis, where practitioners in the community must be used, and where training programs must be simple and cost-efficient (effectiveness research). While effectiveness research is in its infancy the existing data generated thus far support the use of EBT in clinical practice (Wade, Treat, & Stuart, 1998; Sanderson, Raue, & Wetzler, 1999; Franklin, Abramowitz, & Kozac, 2000; Tuschen-Caffier, Pook, & Frank, 2001; Antonuccio, Thomas, & Danton, 1997; Otto, Pollack, & Maki, 2000). Nevertheless, much research remains to be done to modify treatment manuals and training procedures. For example, treatment manuals must be modified to take into account comorbid diagnoses. In addition, training procedures used in efficacy studies must be modified to improve their efficiency and then the validity of streamlined training needs to be determined. This work is underway and will have considerable relevance to the psychotherapy training of practitioners in the future.

## IV. An Overview of Evidence-Based Psychotherapy

Comprehensive reviews exist which have identified psychotherapies that have been specified in a manual, have specific criteria for training and competence evaluations, and have supporting data from controlled clinical trials (*e.g.*, Chambless *et al.*, 1998; Nathan & Gorman, 1998; Weissman *et al.*, 2000). Chambless and Ollendick (2001) recently completed the most extensive review in that they integrated the efforts of eight workgroups (from the U.S., U.K., & Canada) focused on identifying empirically supported psychotherapies. Although the criteria used to define EBT were not the same for each workgroup, overall, the criteria used tended to be conservative. For a treatment to be defined as empirically supported by any of the workgroups, support from at least one rigorous randomized clinical trial was necessary.

Based upon Chambless and Ollendick's (2001) "review of reviews" it is accurate to say that at least one evidence-based treatment (and sometimes several) exist for the full spectrum of psychiatric disorders including:

**Anxiety and Stress**

Agoraphobia/panic disorders with agoraphobia

Blood injury phobia

Generalized anxiety disorder

Geriatric Anxiety

Obsessive-compulsive disorder

Panic disorder

Post-traumatic stress disorder

Public speaking anxiety

Social anxiety/phobia

Specific Phobia

**Chemical Abuse and Dependence**

Alcohol abuse and dependence

Benzodiazepine withdrawal

Cocaine abuse

Opiate Dependence

**Depression**

Bipolar disorder

Geriatric Depression

Major Depression

**Other Disorders**

Anorexia

Binge-eating disorder

Borderline personality disorder

Bulimia

Chronic Pain

Irritable-bowel syndrome

Marital Discord

Migraine Headache

Obesity

Schizophrenia

Smoking Cessation

Sexual Dysfunction

*(Because of space limitations, many other less common disorders have been left off; see Chambless & Ollendick (2001) for a complete list).*

Evidence-based psychotherapies are not efficacious for all conditions (for example, interpersonal psychotherapy has been shown to be ineffective in two clinical trials with opiate abusers). However, for several disorders, psychotherapies have been shown to be as effective as psychotropic interventions (*e.g.*, panic disorder, major depression, bulimia-nervosa). Thus, having psychotherapy available as an alternative to medication is important for patients who do not want to take medication (*e.g.*, pregnant or lactating women), who cannot tolerate medications (*e.g.*, side-effects, adverse reactions), as well as for patients who are not responsive to medications. For other disorders, psychotherapy is an invaluable adjunct (but not a solo treatment) to medication (*e.g.*, bipolar disorder, schizophrenia), enhancing medication compliance, reducing residual symptoms, and decreasing relapse.

In this section we highlight data on the efficacy of specific EBT for several commonly occurring psychiatric disorders.

Depression. Both IPT (Weissman *et al.*, 1979; Elkin *et al.*, 1989) and CBT (cf. Glaoguen, Cottraux, & Cucherat, 1998; Elkin *et al.*, 1989) have been shown to be as effective in reducing symptoms as psychotropic medication for acute treatment of major depression (Depression Guideline Panel, 1993). However, the onset of action is slower for psychotherapy. An amalgam of CBT and IPT (cognitive behavioral-analysis system of psychotherapy) has been shown to be effective in the treatment of chronic depression, and when combined with medication, increased the response rate from 55% to 85% (Keller *et al.*, 2000).

Depression is associated with a high relapse rate. When administered less intensively (approximately once a month) following an acute phase of weekly treatment, both IPT and CBT have been shown to decrease the rate of relapse and recurrences (Frank *et al.*, 1990; Jarrett *et al.*, 1998).

Although not as extensive, controlled trials have also supported the use of IPT and CBT for the treatment of adolescent depression (Brent *et al.*, 1997; Rosello & Bernal, 1998; Mufson *et al.*, 1994, 1999) and late-life depression (Sloane *et al.*, 1985; Reynolds *et al.*, 1999).

Psychotherapy has also been shown to be an efficacious treatment for depression secondary to other problems. For example, IPT has been shown to reduce depression for depressed HIV-positive patients (Markowitz *et al.*, 1995), and both IPT and CBT have been shown to be effective in reducing depression in patients with marital dysfunction (O'Leary & Beach, 1990; Foley *et al.*, 1989).

Bipolar Disorder. IPT and CBT for bipolar disorder target: 1) social/interpersonal events that may be triggers or consequences of bipolar episodes (*e.g.*, interpersonal disputes) and/or 2) mediating mechanisms (such as distorted cognitions, disrupted circadian rhythms). A social rhythm regulation component was added to standard IPT (Interpersonal and Social Rhythm Therapy – IPSRT) to address the specific issues in treating bipolar patients (Frank, Kupfer, Ehlers *et al.*, 1994; Basco & Rush, 1995; Miklowitz & Goldstein, 1997). These treatments are considered adjuncts in combination with medication (e.g., Lam, Bright, Jones *et al.*, 2000). The effectiveness of these psychotherapies in combination with medication for bipolar disorder is currently being tested in a large-scale, multi-site study.

**Anxiety Disorders.** Treatment manuals based upon the principles of CBT exist for each of the anxiety disorders and include several common components: psychoeducation, cognitive restructuring, relaxation strategies, and exposure procedures. These strategies are tailored to address the specific psychopathology associated with each disorder.

There is a considerable body of evidence from controlled studies supporting the efficacy of CBT for the range of anxiety disorders (cf. Nathan & Gorman, 1998 for a comprehensive review): agoraphobia (*e.g.*, Chambless, Foa, Groves, & Goldstein, 1979), generalized anxiety disorder (*e.g.*, Barlow, Rapee, & Brown, 1992), obsessive-compulsive disorder (*e.g.*, Fals-Stewart, Marks, & Schafer, 1993), panic disorder (*e.g.*, Barlow, Gorman, Shear, & Woods, 2000), social phobia (*e.g.*, Heimberg, Liebowitz, Hope, *et al.*, 1998), and posttraumatic stress disorder (*e.g.*, Foa, Rothbaum, Riggs, & Murdock, 1991).

**Schizophrenia.** Efficacy studies of psychotherapy for schizophrenia typically compare two or more treatments in patients who are also receiving antipsychotic medication. Psychotherapy is seen as an adjunct to medication. The focus of outcome is relapse prevention rather than symptom reduction at post-treatment. EBT of schizophrenia can best be viewed as attempts to decrease the patient's vulnerability to relapse by remediating deficits (*e.g.*, social skills training); increasing medication compliance (*e.g.*, providing patients with skills to discuss side-effects with their doctor rather than just discontinuing medication); and reducing stress in the family (*e.g.*, decreasing expressed emotion, providing problem-solving strategies for resolving family conflicts).

Social skills training can lower relapse rates in patients with schizophrenia. In a study by Hogarty, Anderson, and Reiss (1986), patients being treated with medication who received social skills training had a significantly lower relapse rate than those who received individual supportive psychotherapy (20% vs 41%). Overall, when compared to treatment as usual, behavioral, supportive, and systems based family intervention strategies were efficacious in reducing relapse rates in patients with schizophrenia (*e.g.*, Falloon, Boyd, & McGill, 1984; Leff *et al.*, 1985; Schooler *et al.*, 1997). The efficacy of the various family interventions (behavioral, supportive, & systems) appear to be equivalent (Baucom, Shoham, Mueser, Daiuto, & Stickle, 1998). Indeed, the only direct comparison of two evidence-based family interventions found that supportive family therapy and behavioral family therapy were not significantly different. These findings are not surprising considering the family intervention strategies across the three theoretical orientations share many common essential treatment components (Baucom *et al.*, 1998). There is evidence that family therapy involving the use of insight-oriented techniques and focusing on the past is not beneficial in reducing relapse (Kottgen, Sonnichsen, Mollenhauer, & Jurth, 1984) and can be associated with negative outcomes (McFarlane, Link *et al.*, 1995).

## Description of Two Evidence-Based Psychotherapies

There are a variety of psychotherapies that have been shown to be efficacious for at least one disorder. However, most are variants or modifications of two modes of psychotherapy– interpersonal therapy (IPT) and cognitive behavior therapy (CBT) which have had the most testing.

<u>Cognitive Behavioral Therapy.</u> CBT is based upon the premise that emotional disorders stem from distorted, negative thoughts (cognitions) and maladaptive behaviors. The theoretical and empirical sources of CBT based on a cognitive model of emotional disorder and on learning theory have been discussed elsewhere (Beck *et al.*, 1979; Beck, Emery, Greenberg, 1985; Lewinsohn *et al.*, 1986). CBT utilizes strategies to change cognitions (*e.g.*, to reduce harsh self-criticism that may lead to depression, and catastrophizing about events that may lead to anxiety) and behaviors (*e.g.*, decrease phobic avoidance, increase assertiveness) related to the patient's psychopathology. While cognitive and behavioral methods are aimed at different psychopathological processes, in fact they have an overlapping effect (*i.e.*, cognitive methods may produce a change in behavior, and behavioral methods may produce a change in cognition). Thus, in CBT, the therapist focuses directly on modifying thoughts and behaviors. CBT is relatively brief (usually four to eight weeks) and CBT differs from traditional forms of psychotherapy in the following ways:

1. ***A focus on symptoms.*** The goal is to improve the patient's quality of life and restore social and occupational functioning by remediating symptoms that the patient and therapist mutually agree upon as problematic.

2. ***An emphasis on the present and future***. In CBT the therapist works to help patients deal more effectively with problems or symptoms that they are currently experiencing, as opposed to examining their early childhood.

3. ***Explicit, ongoing assessment***. In order to assess for progress (or lack thereof), symptoms are evaluated throughout treatment using objective patient and/or therapist rating scales, thus increasing the therapists' accountability.

4. ***A high level of therapist activity***. In addition to structuring the sessions and maintaining the symptom focused direction, the therapist is responsible for introducing and implementing systematic cognitive and behavioral strategies which will allow the patient to change his/her distorted cognitions and maladaptive behaviors.

5. ***An emphasis on generalizing therapy skills***. In CBT, progress depends largely upon the patient's use of time outside the therapy session. Therefore, every effort is made to facilitate the transfer of learning from the session to the patient's environment (e.g., patients are initially given "homework assignments" to carry out between sessions). Theoretically, if patients use the techniques introduced in session to reduce emotional distress outside of the session, the techniques will be reinforcing to the patient, and thus, continue to be utilized. Thus, in CBT patients are empowered to cope with their problems, and dependence upon the therapist is minimized.

Interpersonal Psychotherapy (IPT). IPT was first developed as a time-limited based treatment for depression by Klerman *et al.*, 1984, and has been subsequently modified to deal with different types of mood and non-mood disorders (see Weissman *et al.*, 2000 for an update). The theoretical and empirical source is based on Bowley's attachment theory and the body of research showing the relationship between loss of attachment, stressful life events and development of symptoms (Klerman *et al.*, 1984). These clinical findings are now under investigation using modern techniques of neuroscience such as studies on the long-lasting effects of stress exposure on physiology, brain structure, function, and a growing body of animal research on behavioral and biological effects on potent stressors occurring at specific points in development (Costello *et al.*, In press). The basic premise of IPT is that, irrespective of their cause, psychiatric disorders usually occur within a social and interpersonal context. Thus, in IPT therapists teach patients to understand the relationship between the onset and fluctuation of their symptoms and current problems and to find ways of dealing with their interpersonal problems. IPT treatments differ from traditional forms of psychotherapy in a number of ways as follows:

1. ***Time-limited and focused***. IPT is time limited, usually eight to 12 weeks: weekly sessions or monthly in case of maintenance treatment. After the initial diagnostic evaluation, which involves systematic assessment and is discussed openly with the patient, the patient and therapist agree on one or two areas of focus. The therapist focuses on one or two problem areas in the patient's current interpersonal functioning (grief, role disputes, transitions, role deficits).

2. ***An emphasis on current interpersonal relationships***. While a brief review of the patient's past relationships and interactions does occur (to enhance the therapist's understanding of the patient's patterns of interpersonal relationships), the focus of the sessions is on the patient's current social functioning.

3. ***Interpersonal instead of intrapsychic***. In IPT, the therapist does not attempt to see the current situation as a manifestation of an internal conflict. Instead, the patient's behavior is explored in terms of disputes in interpersonal relationships.

4. ***Personality is recognized, but not focused on***. While personality is considered important and is believed to affect several aspects of treatment (e.g., outcome, patient-therapist relationship), in IPT the therapist does not explicitly set out to alter the patient's personality. It should be noted that one exception to this is in IPT for Borderline Personality Disorder - but even here, the patient is not confronted directly.

5. ***A moderate level of therapist activity***. The therapist acts as an ally, and fosters the patient's positive expectations about the therapeutic relationship. The therapeutic relationship is not seen as a reenactment of the patient's previous relationships with others, and the therapist may use both reassurance and direct advice whenever they seem most helpful (but generally keeps

them to a minimum in order to foster the patient's own sense of competence). The therapist can also be selectively self-revealing in interactions with the patient and, when relevant to the issues at hand, may express personal opinions or give brief examples of problems from his or her own life. While the therapist does not assign formal homework, homework is implicit in solving focal interpersonal problems during time-limited treatment. As with CBT, the emphasis is on planning and preparing the patient to make (interpersonal) changes in life outside of the therapist's office.

## V. Learning Evidence-Based Treatment

Results of our efforts to learn about current educational curriculum, training and continuing education as it pertains to psychotherapy will be presented. Clearly, a comprehensive review is needed.

In principle, the majority of providers of psychotherapy (*i.e.*, social workers, psychologists, and psychiatrists) would probably agree on the necessity of providing empirical support for their interventions. The public expects to receive an effective treatment from these licensed professionals. Hence, one would expect that training programs would embrace evidence-based treatments. However, we will show that one major obstacle to the use of evidenced-based treatments is their near absence in many training programs for psychologists and social workers and in residency training programs for psychiatrists. This lag may be due in part to the recency of the evidence, although some is due to ideologic differences. Training efforts are more vigorous in Canada, Great Britain, Holland, Iceland, Germany and Spain where calls for workshops, individual training and supervision in EBT by psychiatrists, general practitioners (in Canada) and psychologists have been overwhelming. This view is based on personal experience and not systematic survey.

### Residency and Graduate Training

**Psychiatrists.** Accreditation criteria for psychiatry residency programs set forth by the Accreditation Council for Graduate Medical Education (2000) do not emphasize training in evidence-based psychotherapy but are further along than the other professions in that CBT will be included in the new accreditation criteria. The psychotherapy criteria emphasize training toward competency in brief therapy, cognitive-behavioral therapy, combined psychotherapy and psychopharmacology, psychodynamic therapy, and supportive therapy. Thus, manualized evidence-based psychotherapies, such as those identified in clinical practice guidelines, are not emphasized and psychotherapy that has not been subjected to clinical trials testing is included. According to Dr. Lisa Mellman (personal communication, 7/2/01) who is a member of the American Association of Directors of Psychiatry Residency Training, the plan is to continue to move in the direction of defining and standardizing competency criteria rather than emphasizing training in specific psychotherapies. This approach has some value in that general therapeutic skills will be emphasized. With this background learning manualized psychotherapy is considerably easier if such a mechanism to do so was in place. We could not find any surveys of actual residency training practice in psychiatry. It will be interesting to see how these new criteria are implemented.

**Psychologists.** Guidelines set forth by the Committee on Accreditation (1996) of the American Psychological Association state that training should be based upon "the science of psychology" but allow programs to state their own "philosophy of training." As a result, programs may choose to ignore evidence-based approaches that are not consistent with their philosophy of training. The guideline does not mention training in manualized, evidence-based approaches as a priority, although it does note that "students should be trained in implementing intervention strategies (including training in empirically supported procedures)." Thus, while there is mention of scientifically evaluated treatments, overall, the document is vague and does not emphasize the importance of training in the specific empirically supported approaches defined above.

One would expect psychologists to be particularly receptive to EBTs since a large portion of the development and testing of these treatments was initiated by psychologists. However, a survey of clinical psychology doctoral programs and internship programs revealed that training in most EBTs is lacking (Crits-Christoph, Frank, Chambless, Brody, & Karp, 1995).

For example, two of the first-line treatments for depression listed by the AHCPR Depression Treatment Guideline, CBT and IPT, are not universally taught in graduate and internship training. Specifically, among clinical psychology *internship* programs - the place where clinical psychologists receive the bulk of supervised clinical experience – only 59% of programs provided supervision in CBT for depression, and a mere 8% of programs provided supervision in IPT. University *doctoral* programs were somewhat better, with 80% offering supervision in CBT and 16% in IPT.

Having supervision available does not mean that students are required to receive it. As a result, these numbers do not indicate that 80% of students are, in fact, receiving training in cognitive therapy. For example, based upon personal experience as a faculty member at Rutgers University, although training in cognitive therapy for depression is available, only about one-quarter of the students seek supervision in this modality. Thus, the percentages are likely an overestimation of the total number of clinical psychology students actually receiving training in these approaches.

If one examines the training in EBTs for other disorders, the numbers are even lower (Crits-Christoph *et al.*, 1995). For example, the survey revealed that only 22% of adult-focused internship sites provide supervision in IPT for bulimia and only 3% required it, 14% (2% required) in CBT for social phobia, 22% (4% required) in Exposure/Response Prevention for OCD, 25% (3% required) in family education programs for schizophrenia, 26% (4% required) in exposure treatment for phobias, and 54% (8% required) in CBT for panic disorder.

The numbers reflecting psychotherapy training students receive in graduate school are not very different from internship training: 21% provide supervision in IPT for bulimia, 19% in CBT for social phobia, 48% in Exposure/Response Prevention for OCD, 22% in family education programs for schizophrenia, 59% in exposure treatment for phobias, and 70% in CBT for panic disorder. (The survey did not ask doctoral programs to note if they <u>required</u> the treatment, thus those data are not available, but as noted above, the actual number of students receiving training in these approaches is likely to be considerably lower).

Since most of these treatments represent a first-line intervention for the respective disorder (with some of the treatments being the <u>only</u> empirically supported psychotherapy, such as exposure/response prevention for OCD), it is not as though training in that approach is being eschewed because of training in another evidence-based approach.

<u>**Social Workers**</u>. The Educational Policy from the Council on Social Work Education (1999) does not prescribe any particular curriculum for psychotherapy or counseling (Mullen, personal communication, 2001). Students are expected to become competent and effective practitioners and to evaluate research studies and apply relevant

findings to their practice. There are no guidelines on including empirically based approaches in the training. Since most clinical training occurs through fieldwork, it is unlikely that students receive any training in EBTs. We could not find data on actual training in EBT or on the use of guidelines in social work graduate programs. However, the writing of Mullen & Bacon, both social workers, on the adoption and implementation of evidence-based effective treatments and quality control in social work practice are relevant (Mullen & Bacon, In press-a and b). They conducted a pilot survey of a large urban voluntary mental health/social service agency, which they stated was known for its quality of services and training. While social workers were the main providers of service, the staff included psychiatrists and psychologists. The sample survey was small (N=124) and the response rate poor so results must be viewed cautiously. A survey of a large sample of social workers that are members of the national organization is underway. In light of the absence of other data, the preliminary observations drawn by the authors are interesting. The authors focused on practice guidelines as they believed these were central to the implementation of EBT.

The three mental health professions represented in this survey were strikingly different in their knowledge of practice guidelines and EBT. Psychiatrists were relatively well informed whereas social workers were poorly informed, typically not even aware of the existence of practice guidelines. Psychologists were somewhere in-between. Once told what practice guidelines were, social workers were inclined to be open to their use. Social workers generally were not using research findings or research methods in their practice. Psychiatrists and to a lesser extent psychologists were using findings and methods of assessment. Many social workers did not read the research literature or even other professional literature. Psychiatrists read this literature frequently. Social workers were heavy users of consultation, much more so than the other professionals who functioned more autonomously. Social workers frequently sought guidance from supervisors and other consultants who were viewed as repositories of knowledge based on experience. Given the low use of research methods and infrequent reading of professional literature, Mullen & Bacon conclude that it is unlikely that social work practitioners will be influenced significantly through these routes. Rather, supervisors and consultants seem to be the most promising conduit for knowledge regarding practice guidelines and other forms of evidence-based practice for social workers. Social workers appear to be open to guidelines so long as they are perceived as helping to improve practice, but their preference is for guidelines that represent professional consensus rather than research evidence. A few social work practitioners deviated from this norm, appearing to function more autonomously through behaviors similar to those of the psychiatrists in the sample. These social workers expressed preference for evidence-based guidelines and they had higher frequencies of reading research articles and professional publications. They concluded that these social workers may be important resources for dissemination of evidence-based practice knowledge within social work organizations. It is likely that their training has provided them with research skills relevant to practice. These findings, they conclude, have implications for technologies needed to assist practitioners in identification and use of evidence-based guidelines; for quality control and accountability; and for education.

**Continuing Education.** No formal process exists to disseminate and train practitioners in the use of EBTs (Calhoun, Moras, Pilkonis, & Rehm, 1998). Clinicians trained ten years ago are unlikely to be up-to-date with the newer, evidence-based psychotherapies, since the data supporting EBTs have appeared in the past 10 to 15 years. Continuing Education (CE) Programs have the potential to fill this void.

Workshops are given on EBT at the annual national meetings of psychiatrists and psychologists. Periodically CE workshops outside the professional organizations are offered. However, none of the mental health groups require updated training in EBT. The decision is left to the individual. There is no way to insure the transfer of these treatments to established practitioners or to set standards or monitor quality. Since experienced clinicians are already overworked by changes in healthcare delivery they may feel negative about yet another requirement, time burden or a possible restriction in practice.

Other obstacles to updated training exist. While there is a dearth of information on this topic, those that exist are primarily limited to psychologists but may apply to social workers and psychiatrists. For the most part practicing psychologists tend not to believe that evidence-based treatments (and related procedures such as practice guidelines, structured or validated assessment procedures) are useful in their clinical practice (Addis & Krasnow, 2000; Plante *et al.*, 1999). The most frequent reasons stated are that EBT limits creativity and does not take individual patient needs into account.

## VI. Implications in the Evolving Health Care System

The gap in the transfer of EBTs from research to clinical practitioners will impact on the viability of psychotherapy as the healthcare system evolves. The National MEPS data presented above show a decrease in visits for psychotherapy and a dramatic increase in the use of psychotropic medication (see Appendix). The increasing penetration of managed care and the proliferation of clinical practice guidelines and treatment consensus statements have raised the stakes for accountability. The failure to train practitioners in EBT so that they are available to the general public may lead to the disappearance of psychotherapy as a treatment despite data supporting its efficacy.

Managed Care. Managed care organizations (or any other system monitoring the utilization and cost of service such as HMOs, capitated contracts with providers, etc.) are reshaping the practice of psychotherapy. In the traditional fee-for-service model, decisions about the cost and length of treatment were primarily functions of choices made by the doctor and patient, with the allocation of resources (*i.e.*, cost of psychotherapy) being of less concern to the clinician. In fact, the fee-for-service model encouraged the provision of service, as more service created more income. However, in response to the increased costs of psychotherapy and, in particular, to the perceived "endless" nature of psychotherapy, managed care organizations are pressuring clinicians to allocate decreasing amounts of service.

To date, the focus of managed care organizations' cost cutting has been almost entirely on limiting the number of sessions a patient receives. However, in order to compete, managed care organizations will also have to focus on the quality (effectiveness) of psychotherapy, as they strive to satisfy both the consumer (*i.e.*, patient), and payer (*e.g.*, employer providing health benefits). In essence, managed care organizations must balance their motivation to cut costs with effective clinical outcomes. Simply reducing the length of treatment may not accomplish this goal and lead in turn to both consumer dissatisfaction and increased costs down the road (as the severity of the disorder may increase and become less responsive to treatment). Thus, concern for the effectiveness of an intervention will eventually temper the managed care organizations' focus on economics. Ultimately, managed care organizations will be interested in clinicians providing the "optimal intervention: ...the least extensive, intensive, intrusive and costly intervention capable of successfully addressing the presenting problem." (Bennett, 1992).

Clinical Practice Guidelines. Clinical practice guidelines and treatment consensus statements have also impacted upon the practice of psychotherapy. As noted by Smith and Hamilton (1994) "Guidelines are now being developed because there is a perception that inappropriate medical care is sometimes provided and that such inappropriate care has both health and economic consequences" (p. 42). Guidelines are developed to ensure that patients uniformly receive the optimal intervention (whether it is a type of medication, surgical procedure, or psychotherapeutic intervention).

The Agency for Healthcare Policy and Research (AHCPR) within the Public Health Service is a federal agency involved in clinical guideline development. Only treatments with documented efficacy from randomized controlled trials are emphasized. As a result, the recommendations of the clinical practice guidelines are quite clear. For example, consider the wording from the AHCPR guideline for Depression (Depression Guideline Panel, 1993), which states that, "[when psychotherapy is to be selected as the sole treatment], the psychotherapy should generally be time-limited, focused on current problems, and aimed at symptom resolution rather than personality change as the initial target. Since it has not been established that all forms of psychotherapy are equally effective in major depressive disorder, if one is chosen as the sole treatment, it should have been studied in randomized controlled trials." In addition to endorsing specific treatments for depression that have sufficient empirical evidence (*e.g.*, cognitive behavioral therapy [CBT] and interpersonal psychotherapy [IPT]), the report goes on to state: "Long-term therapies are not currently indicated as first-line acute phase treatments" (p.84).

Consensus statements are also influential in determining which treatments should be delivered. In 1991, a Consensus Development Conference on the Treatment of Panic Disorder sponsored by the National Institute of Mental Health and the Office of Medical Applications of Research, National Institutes of Health was held. The available scientific evidence from clinical trials determined the merit of various treatments (Wolf & Maser, 1994). A number of specific treatments were judged to be effective for panic disorder, including several pharmacological compounds and CBT (cf., Panic Consensus Statement published in Wolf & Maser, 1994). The Panic Consensus

Statement is clearly negative on the use of treatments not supported by empirical evidence. "One risk of maintaining individuals in non-validated treatments of panic disorder is that misplaced confidence in the therapy's potential effectiveness may preclude application of more effective treatment." The statement also spells out a specific concern about the use of psychotherapies without demonstrated effectiveness for panic disorder: "The nature of the therapeutic relationship makes it difficult for the patient to seek additional or alternate treatment."

As clinical guidelines and treatment consensus statements continue to emerge for a wide array of emotional disorders, they will have a significant impact upon the way clinicians practice psychotherapy. In effect, these documents set standards of care which, if ignored, leave the clinician both ethically and legally vulnerable. Health insurance companies and managed care plans are now providing their practitioners with copies of guidelines and asking that they be followed. For example, Merit Behavioral Care Corporation, in a letter to their providers (July 14, 1997), stated the following: "Consistent with national standards, the Medical Affairs Committee of MBC endorses clinical practice guidelines." They then provided references to specific treatment guidelines created by the American Psychiatric Association for schizophrenia, major depression, substance abuse, and bipolar disorder.

Managed care and clinical practice guidelines are placing increasing pressure to deliver psychotherapies that are cost-effective and empirically supported (Sanderson, 1995). Practitioners have not been concerned about scientific testing and accountability. As practice guidelines become the "standard of care," accountability will be essential. Ultimately, treatments without supporting efficacy data are less likely to be reimbursed (Trabin, 1994).

## VII. Recommendations

This review has highlighted the progress in the specification of psychotherapy including an emphasis on time-limited treatment; development of training procedures for research; and their testing in controlled clinical trials. As a result, there is an increasing availability of evidence-based psychotherapy and an increased recommendation for their use in official guidelines and within the managed health-care industry.

Clinical practice also is changing. While the number of persons seeking psychotherapy has not changed over the last decade, the course of treatment tends to be shorter and there has been an increase in psychotherapy provided by social workers. Unfortunately, the three mental health professional groups (psychiatrists, psychologists and social workers) who provide most of the psychotherapy have received little training in EBT, with social workers having the least exposure. As a result, there is a substantial gap between research evidence, clinical practice and graduate training in these treatments. Furthermore, there is no mandate for continuing education in EBT for practicing professionals. While workshops in EBT are held at professional meetings, their quality and content are not monitored. They are voluntary and there are no procedures for follow-up or credentialing participants. Ironically, social workers, the group that has played an increased role in providing psychotherapy during the past decade is the least likely to have training in evidence-based procedures. Thus, the gap between research and practice does not appear to be decreasing with the accumulating body of literature and proliferation of treatment guidelines. The following are our preliminary recommendations to begin to close the gap between research and the practice of psychotherapy.

**Recommendation #1.**

There is a dearth of information on the specific content of psychotherapy training within residency (psychiatry) and graduate (psychology, social work) training programs. As a first step, we recommend that an in-depth study be conducted to determine what is currently included in the respective residency and graduate training programs. What is required of trainees and what is actually achieved? Is training in EBT part of the program? If so, what is the nature and quality of this training? In order to accomplish this, program heads, faculty members, and students/residents should be surveyed to have a clear understanding of the content of training from multiple vantage points.

**Recommendation #2.**

While there have been reviews of efficacy studies in psychotherapy, the field is moving ahead rapidly and thus there need to be regular, systematic evaluations of the literature to determine the latest evidence-based psychotherapeutic treatments. In addition, none of the reviews to date have been conducted with a view towards improving training or dissemination of EBT. Few studies have systematically catalogued the training and experience of the mental health professionals providing the treatment within the study. Therefore, we recommend that efficacy and effectiveness studies should be reviewed to determine the current status of EBTs. What is the state of the evidence? Have efficacy studies been replicated? How many treatments have effectiveness studies supporting their use in the field? What work is in progress? What is the level of education and training of the therapists? What is the nature of the training utilized for therapists in research studies?

**Recommendation #3.**

With information gathered from Recommendations 1 and 2 as a background, we recommend that key decision makers in residency training and graduate programs, deans, department chairs, training directors, representatives from national health care organizations and consumer groups be assembled to review the data and develop policy and strategies for implementation. Perhaps the independent Institute of Medicine (IOM) could convene this group to review the data and develop a consensus as to steps needed to implement training in EBT, including plans for training material and a model curriculum.

**Recommendation #4.**

Policy about CE requirements should focus on developing continuing education requirements in EBT for professionals. The following questions must be addressed. What format should the training include? What competency requirements and credentialing are needed? These decisions need the involvement of major professional organizations as well as the national and international organizations that have emerged around the leading EBTs (*e.g.*, The Academy of Cognitive Therapy and the International Society for Interpersonal Psychotherapy are developing competency criteria).

**Recommendation #5.**

While the actual core curriculum for training in EBT will need to be determined by each discipline, in addition to training in the clinical application of EBTs, a core curriculum should include information on the method for systematic assessment of the patient's signs, symptoms and diagnosis (*e.g.*, use of reliable and valid symptom rating scales); information on how treatments are tested so that practitioners can evaluate the validity of new treatments as they emerge; information on how treatment manuals are developed;

the indications and contraindications for the various EBTs; current treatment guidelines so that clinicians know what treatments are recommended by expert panels; and current efficacy data so that clinicians can learn to evaluate the quality and strength of the supporting studies. For the non-medical clinician, information on psychotropic medication and indications for referrals for evaluation and treatment should be included.

Some attention should be given to specialty psychotherapy training in residency and graduate training programs. For example, a psychiatry resident interested in molecular genetics, a social work student in community action or a psychology student in experimental testing may get an introduction to content whereas trainees who specialize in patient/client treatment would get more intense training and supervision in EBT.

We realize that mental health specialty is only a portion of social work practice. However, social workers come into contact with large numbers of people who have comorbid mental health problems where appropriate identification and possible referral for treatment may be most useful. The amount of psychotherapy provided by social workers is increasing and we expect this trend will continue. Yet social workers have the least training in evidence-based procedures. In light of these trends we recommend that special attention be given to social work education.

**Recommendation #6.**

With regard to actual training, we recommend that the general core therapeutic skills of EBT continue to be taught in residency and graduate programs. This content is only informally taught in social work graduate school during supervision. Therefore, the content and quality of social work supervision needs to be reviewed and some shortening of fieldwork might accommodate the new material. Once core evidence-based psychotherapy skills have been taught, training in specific EBTs should be initiated, especially for commonly occurring disorders. In order to accomplish this, it makes sense to follow the training procedures developed for research protocols. These include reading the manuals, didactic review of material, and case supervision using video or audiotapes. In light of the psychotherapy recommendations from a variety of independent clinical practice guidelines, we tentatively recommend that the core training include CBT and IPT. Training in the various adaptations of these treatments, as well as other specific behavioral techniques, family interventions, and group methods could be added for practitioners who want to specialize in psychotherapy.

## VIII. Concluding Comments

We realize that this new material may appear to overburden already compact training programs and will require some modification of current training. Also, clinicians already dealing with the restrictions on their practice may find these recommendations just another added burden. We also realize that the gap is in part due to the recency of the data and to the many pressures training programs have had to deal with as a result of the changing health care environment. However, findings such as those by Goisman *et al.* (1999) showing that the use of evidence based procedures have not increased over a ten-year period, despite a substantial amount of supporting data and the proliferation of treatment guidelines, are quite disappointing and suggest that a more deliberate intervention is necessary if we are going to close the gap between research and practice. Moreover, the increased penetration of managed care and the proliferation of guidelines will increase accountability. The failure to increase EBT and to train clinicians so that these treatments are available to the public could lead to the disappearance of psychotherapy as a treatment.

## Acknowledgements

The authors appreciate the help of Drs. Lisa Mellman, Ronald Reider, Edward Mullen and Mark Olfson, who provided information on training and clinical practice and Marc Gameroff who analyzed the Medical Expenditure Panel Survey data and prepared the Appendix for this paper. All are from Columbia University. We have tried to be as objective as possible in presenting our views but since our backgrounds could color our views we want to openly describe them. William Sanderson is trained in clinical psychology; is on the psychology faculty at Rutgers University and has a private practice. Myrna Weissman is trained as a social worker and an epidemiologist; is on the psychiatry and public health faculty at Columbia University and is a developer of interpersonal psychotherapy. She does not have a private practice.

## References

Accreditation Council for Graduate Medical Education. (September 2000). *Psychiatry.* Http:www.acgme.org

Addis, M.E. & Krasnow, A.D. (2000). A national survey of practicing psychologists' attitudes toward psychotherapy treatment manuals. *Journal of Consulting and Clinical Psychology,* 68: 333-345.

Antonuccio, D.A., Thomas, M., & Danton, W.G. (1997). A cost-effectiveness analysis of cognitive behavior therapy and fluoxetine in the treatment of depression. *Behavior Therapy,* 28: 187-210.

Barlow, D.H., Gorman, J.M., Shear, M.K., Woods, S.W. (2000). Cognitive-behavioral therapy, imipramine, and their combination in panic disorder. *Journal of the American Medical Association,* 283: 2529-2536.

Barlow, D.H., Rapee, R., & Brown, T. (1992). Behavioral treatment of generalized anxiety disorder. *Behavior Therapy,* 23: 551-570.

Basco, M.R. & Rush, A.J. Compliance with pharmacotherapy in mood disorders. *Psychiatric Annals,* 25: 269-270.

Baucom, D.H., Shoham, V., Mueser, K.T., Daiuto, A.D., Stickle, T.R. (1998). Empirically supported couple and family interventions for marital distress and adult mental health problems. *Journal of Consulting and Clinical Psychology,* 66: 53-88.

Beck, A.T., Emery, G., Greenberg, R.L., (1985). Anxiety Disorders and Phobias: A Cognitive Perspective. New York: Basic Books.

Beck, A.T., Rush, A.J., Shaw, B., Emery, G. (1979). Cognitive Therapy of Depression. New York: Guilford.

Bennett, M.J. (1992). The managed care setting as a framework for clinical practice. In J.L. Feldman and R.J. Fitzpatrick (Eds.), Managed Mental Healthcare: Administrative and Clinical Issues (pp. 203-218). Washington, DC: American Psychiatric Press.

Brent, D.A., Holder, D., Kolko, D., Birmaher, B., Baugher, M., Roth, C. and Johnson, B. (1997). A clinical psychotherapy trial for adolescent depression comparing cognitive, family, and supportive treatments. *Archives of General Psychiatry,* 54: 877-885.

Calhoun, K.S., Moras, K., Pilkonis, P.A. and Rehm, L.P. (1998). Empirically supported treatments: implications for training. *Journal of Consulting and Clinical Psychology,* 66: 151-162.

Chambless, D.L, Baker, M.J., Baucom, D., Beutler, L.E., Calhoun, K.S., Crits-Christoph, P., Daiuto, A., DeRubeis, R., Detweiler, J., Haaga, D.A.F., Johnson, S.B., McCurry, S., Mueser, K.T., Pope, K.S., Sanderson, W.C., Shoham, V., Stickle, T., Williams, D.A., Woody, S.R. (1998). Update on Empirically Validated Therapies: II. *The Clinical Psychologist,* 51: 3-16.

Chambless, D.L., Foa, E.B., Groves, G.A., and Goldstein, A.J. (1979). Flooding with brevital in the treatment of agoraphobia: countereffective? *Behavior Research and Therapy,* 17: 243-251.

Chambless, D.L. and Ollendick, T.H. (2001). Empirically supported psychological interventions: controversies and evidence. *Annual Review of Psychology,* 52: 685-716.

Committee on Accreditation. (2000). Guidelines and principles for accreditation of programs in professional psychology. American Psychological Association.

Costello E.J., Pine D.S., Hammen C., March J.S., Plotsky P.M., Weissman M.M., Biederman J., Goldsmith H.H., Kaufman J., Lewinsohn P.M., Hellander M., Hoagwood K., Koretz D.S., Nelson C.A., Leckman J.F. (In press). Development and natural history of mood disorders. *Biol Psychiatry.*

Crits-Christoph, P., Frank, E., Chambless, D.L., Brody, C. and Karp, J.F. (1995). Training in empirically validated therapies: What are clinical psychology students learning? *Professional Psychology: Research and Practice*, 26: 514-522.

Depression Guideline Panel. (1993). Depression in Primary Care: Volume 2. Treatment of Major Depression. Clinical Practice Guideline, Number 5. Rockville, MD. (Department of Health and Human Services, Public Health Service, Agency for Healthcare Policy and Research. AHCPR Publication No. 93-0551). Washington, DC: US Government Printing Office.

Elkin, I., Shea, M.T., Watkins, J.T., Imber, S.D., Sotsky, S.M., Collins, J.F., Glass, D.R., Pilkonis, P.A., Leber, W.R., Docherty, J.P., Fiester, S.J., & Parloff, M.B. (1989). National Institute of Mental Health treatment of depression collaborative research program. *Archives of General Psychiatry*, 46: 971-982.

Falloon, I.R.H., Boyd, J.L., McGill, C.W., Williamson, M., Razani, J., Moss, J.B., Gilderman, A.M., Simons, G.M. (1985). Family management in the prevention of morbidity in schizophrenia: Clinical outcome of a two year longitudinal study. *Archives of General Psychiatry*, 42: 887-896.

Foa, E.B., Rothbaum, B.O., Riggs, D.S., and Murdock, T.B. (1991). Treatment of post-traumatic stress disorder in rape victims. *Journal of Consulting and Clinical Psychology*, 59: 715-723.

Foley, S.H., Rounsaville, B.J., Weissman, M.M., Sholomskas, D., and Chevron, E. (1989) Individual versus conjoint interpersonal therapy for depressed patients with marital disputes. *International Journal of Family Psychiatry*, 10: 29-42.

Frank, E., Kupfer, D.J., Ehlers, C.L. (1994). Interpersonal and social rhythm therapy for bipolar disorder: integrating interpersonal and behavior approaches. *The Behavior Therapist*, 17: 143-149.

Frank, E., Kupfer, D.J., Perel, J.M., Cornes, C., Jarret, D.B., Mallinger, A.G., Thase, M.E., McEachran, A.B., and Grochocinski, V.J. (1990). Three-year outcomes for maintenance therapies in recurrent depression. *Archives of General Psychiatry*, 47: 1093-1099.

Franklin, M.E., Abramowitz, J.S., Kozak, M.J, Levitt, J.T., and Foa, E.B. (2000). Effectiveness of exposure and response prevention for obsessive-compulsive disorder: Randomized compared with nonrandomized samples. *Journal of Consulting and Clinical Psychology*, 68: 594-602.

Glaoguen, V., Cottraux, J., Cucherat, M. (1998) A meta-analysis of the effects of cognitive therapy in depressed patients. *Journal of Affective Disorders*, 49: 59-72.

Goisman, R.M., Rogers, M.P, Stekettee, G.S., Warshaw, M.G., Cuneo, P., & Keller, M.B. (1993). Utilization of behavioral methods in a multi-center anxiety disorders study. *Journal of Clinical Psychiatry*, 54: 213-218.

Goisman, R.M., Warshaw, M.G., Keller, M.B. (1999). Psychosocial treatment prescriptions for generalized anxiety disorder, panic disorder, and social phobia, 1991-1996. *American Journal of Psychiatry*, 156: 1819-1821.

Heimberg, R.G., Liebowitz, M.R., Hope, D.A., Schneier, F.R., Holt, C.S., Welkowitz, L.A., Juster, H.R., Campeas, R., Bruch, M.A., Cloitre, M., Fallon, B., Klein, D.F. (1998). Cognitive behavioral group therapy vs phenelzine therapy for social phobia. *Archives of General Psychiatry*, 55: 1133-1141.

Hibbs E.D., Jensen P.S. (eds) (1996). Psychological Treatments for Child and Adolescent Disorders: Empirically Based Strategies for Clinical Practice. American Psychological Association Press, Washington, D.C.

Hogarty, G.E., Anderson, C.M., and Reiss, D.J. (1986). Family psychoeducation, social skills training and maintenance chemotherapy in the aftercare treatment of schizophrenia. *Archives of General Psychiatry*, 43: 633-642.

Jarrett, R.B., Basco, M.R., & Risser, R. (1998). Is there a role for continuation phase cognitive therapy for depressed outpatients. *Journal of Consulting and Clinical Psychology,* 66: 1036-1040.

Keller, M.B., McCullough, J.P., Klein, D.N., Arnow, B., Dunner, D.L., Gelenberg, A.J., Markowitz, J.C., Nemeroff, C.B., Russell, J.B., Thase, M.B., Trivedi, M.H., Zajecka, J., Blalock, J.A., Borian, F.E., DeBattista, C., Fawcett, J., Hirschfeld, R.M.A., Jody, D.N., Keitner, G., Kocsis, J.H., Korna, L.M., Kornstein, S.G., Manber, R., Miller, I., Ninan, P., Rothbaum, B., Rush, A.J., Schatzberg, A., Vivian, D. (2000). A comparison of nefazodone, the cognitive behavioral-analysis system of psychotherapy, and their combination in the treatment of chronic depression. *New England Journal of Medicine,* 342: 1462-1470.

Klerman, G.L., Weissman, M.M. & Rounsaville, B.J., Chevron, E. (1984). Interpersonal Psychotherapy for Depression. New York: Basic Books.

Kottgen, C., Sonnichsen, I., Mollenhauer, K., & Jurth, R. (1984). Group therapy with the families of schizophrenic patients: Results of the Hamburg Camberwell Family Interview Study III. *International Journal of Family Psychiatry,* 5: 84-94.

Lam, D.H., Bright, J., Jones, S., Hayward, P., Schuck, N., Chisholm, D., Sham, P. (2000). Cognitive therapy of bipolar illness: A pilot study. *Cognitive Therapy and Research,* 24: 503-520.

Leff, J. Kuipers, L., Berkowitz, R. & Sturgeon, D. (1985). A controlled trial of social intervention in the families of schizophrenic patients: two year follow-up. *British Journal of Psychiatry,* 146: 594-600.

Lewisohn, P.M. (1975). The behavioral study and treatment of depression. In Progress in Behavior Modification, (Eds.) Hersen, M., Eisler, R.M. N.Y. Academic Press, pp. 19-64.

Lewinsohn, P.M., Muñoz, R., Youngren, M., Zeiss, A.M. (1986). Control Your Depression. N.Y: Fireside.

Luborsky L., DeRubeis R.J. (1984). The use of psychotherapy treatment manuals: A small revolution in psychotherapy research styles. *Clinical Psychology Review* 4: 5-14.

Markowitz, J.C., Klerman, G.L., Clougherty, K.F., Spielman, L.A., Jacobsberg, L.B., Fishman, B., Frances, A.J., Kocsis, J.H, & Perry, S. (1995). Individual psychotherapies for depressed HIV-positive patients. *American Journal of Psychiatry,* 152: 1504-1509.

McFarlane, W.R., Link, B., Dushay, R. Marchal, J. and Crilly, J. (1995). Psychoeducational multiple family groups: four-year outcome in schizophrenia. Family Process, 34: 127-144.

Miklowitz, D.J. & Goldstein, M.J. (1997). Bipolar Disorder: A Family Focused Treatment Approach. New York: Guilford Press.

Mufson, L., Weissman M.M., Moreau D. (1999). The efficacy of interpersonal psychotherapy for depressed adolescents. *Archives of General Psychiatry* 56: 573-579.

Mufson, L., Moreau, D., Weissman, M.M., Wickramaratne, P., Martin, J., and Samoilov, A. (1994). Modifications of interpersonal psychotherapy with depressed adolescents: Phase I and II studies. *Journal of the American Academy of Child and Adolescent Psychiatry,* 33: 695-705.

Mullen, E.J. and Bacon, W.F. (In Press-a). Practitioner adoption and implementation of evidence-based effective treatments and issues of quality control. A. Rosen & E. K. Proctor (Eds.). Developing Practice Guidelines for Social Work Interventions: Issues, Methods, and a Research Agenda. New York: Columbia University Press.

Mullen, E.J. and Bacon, W.F. (In Press-b). A survey of practitioner adoption and implementation of evidence-based treatments. [On-line electronic pre-print]. Available: London, UK: National Institute for Social Work, http://www.intsoceval.net/Stockholm/stockholmpapers.htm

Mullen, E.J. & Bacon, W.F. (2000). Practitioner adoption and implementation of evidence-based effective treatments and issues of quality control. Developing Practice Guidelines for Social Work Intervention, May 3-4, St. Louis, MO.

Nathan, P. E., and Gorman, J.M. (Eds.). (1998). A Guide to Treatments that Work. New York: Oxford University Press.

O'Leary, K.D, and Beach, S. (1990). Marital therapy: A viable treatment for depression and marital discord. *American Journal of Psychiatry,* 147: 183-186.

Otto, M.W., Pollack, M.H., & Maki, K.M. (2000). Empirically supported treatments for panic disorder: costs, benefits, and stepped care. *Journal of Consulting and Clinical Psychology,* 68: 556-563.

Pincus, H.A. (1994). Treatment guidelines: risks are outweighed by the benefits. *Behavioral Healthcare Tomorrow,* 4: 40-45.

Plante, T.G., Andersen, E.N., Boccaccini, M.T. (1999). Empirically supported treatments and related contemporary changes in psychotherapy practice: What do clinical ABPPs think. *The Clinical Psychologist,* 52: 23-31.

Reynolds, C.F., Frank, E., Perel, J.M., Imber, S.D., Cornes, C., Miller, M.D., Mazumdar, S., Houck, P.R., Dew, M.A., Stack, J.A., Pollock, B.G., Kupfer, D.J. (1999). Nortriptyline and interpersonal psychotherapy as maintenance therapies for recurrent major depression: A randomized controlled trial in patients older than fifty-nine years. *Journal of the American Medical Association,* 281: 39-45.

Rosello, J. and Bernal, G. (1996). Adopting cognitive behavioral and interpersonal treatment for depressed Puerto Rican adolescents. In Psychosocial Treatment for Child and Adolescent Disorders, Hebbs, E.P. and Jensen, P.S. (Eds), Washington, DC: American Psychiatric Association Press.

Sanderson, W.C. (1995). Can psychological interventions meet the new demands of health care? *American Journal of Managed Care,* 1: 93-98.

Sanderson, W.C., Hiatt, D., and Schwartz, J. (2001). Psychological treatment of panic disorder by managed care providers. Manuscript in preparation.

Sanderson, W.C., Raue, P.J., and Wetzler, S. (1998). The generalizability of cognitive behavior therapy for panic disorder. *Journal of Cognitive Psychotherapy,* 12: 323-330.

Schooler, N.R., Keith, S.J., Severe, J.B., Mathews, S.M., Bellack, A.S., Glick, I.D., Hargreaves, W.A., Kane, J.M, Ninan, P.T., Frances, A., Jacobs, M., Lieberman, J.A., Mance, R., Simpson, G.M., & Woerner, M.G. (1997). Relapse and rehospitalization during maintenance treatment of schizophrenia: The effects of dose reduction and family therapy. *Archives of General Psychiatry,* 54: 453-463.

Shaw, B.F., Elkin, I., Yamaguchi, J., Olmsted, M., Vallis, T.M. (1999). Therapist competence ratings in relation to clinical outcome in cognitive therapy of depression. *Journal of Consulting and Clinical Psychology,* 67: 837-846.

Sloane, R. B., Staples, F. R., & Schneider, L. S. (1985). Interpersonal therapy vs. nortriptyline for depression in the elderly. In G. D. Burrows, T. R. Norman, & L. Denerstein (Eds.), Clinical and pharmacological studies in psychiatric disorders (pp. 344–346). London: John Libby.

Smith, G.R., & Hamilton, G.E. (1994). Treatment guidelines: provider involvement is critical. *Behavioral Healthcare Tomorrow,* 4: 40-45.

Taylor, C.B., King, R., Margraf, J. (1989). Use of medication and in vivo exposure in volunteers for panic disorder research. *American Journal of Psychiatry,* 146: 1423-1426.

Trabin T. (1994). Toward greater accountability for quality: More science, less art? *Behavioral Healthcare Tomorrow,* 3: 1-8.

Tuschen-Caffier, B., Pook, M., & Frank, M. (2001). Evaluation of manual-based cognitive-behavioral therapy for bulimia nervosa in a service setting. *Behaviour Research and Therapy,* 39: 299-308.

Wade, W.A., Treat, T.A., and Stuart, G.L. (1998). Transporting an empirically supported treatment for panic disorder to a service clinic setting: a benchmarking strategy. *Journal of Consulting and Clinical Psychology*, 66: 231-239.

Weissman, M.M., Markowitz, J.C., and Klerman, G.L. (2000). Comprehensive Guide to Interpersonal Therapy. New York: Basic Books.

Weissman, M.M., Prusoff, B.A., DiMascio A, Neu, C, Goklaney, M., Klerman, G.L. (1979). The efficacy of drugs and psychotherapy in the treatment of acute depressive episodes. *American Journal of Psychiatry*, 136: 555-558.

Wolfe, B.E. and Maser, J.D. (1994). Treatment of Panic Disorders: A Consensus Statement. Washington, DC: American Psychiatric Association Press.

Woody, S.R. & Sanderson, W.C. (1998). Manuals for empirically supported treatments: 1998 update from the task force on psychological interventions. *The Clinical Psychologist*, 51: 17-21.

Zastowny, T.R., Lehman, A.F., Cole, R.E., and Kane, C. (1992). Family management of schizophrenia: A comparison of behavioral and supportive family treatment. *Psychiatric Quarterly*, 63: 159-186.

# Appendix:

## *Psychotherapy Use in the U.S. Civilian Non-institutionalized Population in 1987 and 1997*

**Marc J. Gameroff — Myrna M. Weissman**

This appendix presents an analysis comparing psychotherapy usage in the U.S. in 1987 and 1997. The data sources are the Household Components of the 1987 National Medical Expenditure Survey (NMES) and the 1997 Medical Expenditure Panel Survey (MEPS), two national probability surveys conducted by the Agency for Healthcare Research and Quality (AHRQ) on the financing and utilization of health care services in the U.S. Both surveys are designed to provide statistically unbiased estimates of utilization by the civilian non-institutionalized population of the U.S in a single calendar year. NMES was conducted in 1987 only, and MEPS has collected data continuously since 1996. Public use data files for calendar year 1997 were recently released and were used for the current analysis. Detailed information about sampling, survey design, reporting sources, and survey items related to demographics, health status, and health care utilization, are available in print form for NMES (*e.g.*, Cohen, DiGaetano, & Waksberg, 1991; Edwards & Berlin, 1989) and on the World Wide Web for MEPS (*e.g.*, AHRQ, Jan., Feb. 2001). An excellent introduction to MEPS can be accessed at *http://www.meps.ahrq.gov/whatis.htm*.

## ANALYSIS

### Rates of Psychotherapy Use

The percentage of the population receiving psychotherapy in 1987 and 1997 was on average 3.4%, with no significant difference between years (**see Table 1**). However, visiting a medical doctor or

**TABLE 1.**
**Percentage of the Civilian U.S. Population With Psychotherapy Use[a], and Mean Number of Visits Per User, 1987 and 1997**

| Psychotherapy Provider Type[b] | % With Psychotherapy Use | | Mean Number of Visits Per User | |
|---|---|---|---|---|
| | 1987 (*N*=34,459) | 1997 (*N*=32,636) | 1987 (*n*=993) | 1997 (*n*=1,136) |
| Medical doctor (M.D.) | 1.6 | 2.3**** | 4.0 | 3.9 |
| Psychologist | 1.1 | 1.3 | 3.4 | 2.5* |
| Social worker | 0.3 | 0.5* | 0.7 | 1.2 |
| Other non-M.D.[c] | 0.9 | 0.5*** | 2.7 | 1.3** |
| Any provider type | 3.2 | 3.6 | 10.8 | 8.9* |

**Note.** *Figures are national estimates based on weighted data from the 1987 National Medical Expenditures Survey (NMES) and the 1997 Medical Expenditure Panel Survey (MEPS). SUDAAN software was used to account for the complex survey design. Year effects are tested with c2 analysis (% with psychotherapy use; df = 1) or linear regression (mean number of visits per user; df = 1).*

[a] *Psychotherapy users were those who made at least 1 visit to a provider in an office-based practice or a hospital outpatient unit where "psychotherapy/mental health counseling" was the main reason for the visit (NMES) or where "psychotherapy/counseling" was among the services received (MEPS).* [b] *Rows labeled with particular provider types are not mutually exclusive, as a portion of psychotherapy users (16.4% in 1987 and 23.6% in 1997) saw more than 1 provider type.* [c] *The most commonly given titles included: "therapist," "counselor," "mental health counselor," "occupational therapist," "physical therapist," and "nurse/nurse practitioner."*

*$P < .05$. **$P < .01$. ***$P < .001$. ****$P < .0001$. *$P < .05$. **$P < .01$. ***$P < .001$. ****$P < .0001$.

social worker for psychotherapy became more common, and seeing another type of non-M.D. provider became less common. Although the overall "popularity" of psychotherapy did not decrease, those receiving psychotherapy in 1997 had fewer visits. This trend was essentially limited to therapy provided by psychologists and other non-M.D.'s. However, visiting another type of non-M.D. provider was also less common in the population in 1997, while psychologists provided therapy to an equal proportion of the population in 1987 and 1997.

### Rates of Receiving a Psychotropic Medication

While for psychotherapy users the mean number of visits decreased

**TABLE 2.**
**Percentage of the Civilian U.S. Population With At Least One Psychotropic Prescription During the Year, Among Psychotherapy Users[a] and Non-Users, 1987 and 1997**

| Psychotherapy Use and Provider Type[b] | % Receiving Psychotropic Rx 1987 | % Receiving Psychotropic Rx 1997 |
|---|---|---|
| Received psychotherapy… | | |
| …from a medical doctor | 46.5 | 71.4**** |
| …from a psychologist | 24.9 | 47.3**** |
| …from a social worker | 27.6 | 54.2** |
| …from another type of non-M.D.[c] | 24.9 | 52.1**** |
| …from any provider type | 31.2 | 58.1**** |
| Did not receive psychotherapy | 5.5 | 6.8**** |

*Note. Figures are national estimates based on weighted data from the 1987 National Medical Expenditures Survey (NMES) and the 1997 Medical Expenditure Panel Survey (MEPS). SUDAAN software was used to account for the complex survey design. Year effects in this table are tested with c2 analysis (df = 1).*

[a] *Psychotherapy users were those who made at least 1 visit to a provider in an office-based practice or a hospital outpatient unit where "psychotherapy/mental health counseling" was the main reason for the visit (NMES) or where "psychotherapy/counseling" was among the services received (MEPS).*

[b] *Rows labeled with particular provider types are not mutually exclusive, as a portion of psychotherapy users (16.4% in 1987 and 23.6% in 1997) saw more than 1 provider type.*

[c] *The most commonly given titles included: "therapist," "counselor," "mental health counselor," "occupational therapist," "physical therapist," and "nurse/nurse practitioner."*

*$P$ < .05. **$P$ < .01. ***$P$ < .001. ****$P$ < .0001.

between 1987 and 1997, the likelihood of receiving a psychotropic medication almost doubled, from 31% in 1987 to 58% in 1997 (**see Table 2**). Naturally, this trend was pronounced among individuals receiving psychotherapy from medical doctors (47% in 1987 to 71% in 1997), however rates also increased sharply for individuals seeing psychologists, social workers, and other types of non-M.D. providers, from about 25% in 1987 to 50% in 1997. Among those in the population who did not receive psychotherapy, the likelihood of receiving a psychotropic prescription was below 7% in both years but showed a statistically significant increase.

## Demographic Characteristics of Psychotherapy Users

The demographic profile of psychotherapy users in the U.S. did not change considerably between 1987 and 1997 (**see Table 3**). For instance, the ratio of females to males was roughly 3:2, and the racial/ethnic distribution of users was fairly stable within and across

**TABLE 3. Demographic Characteristics of Psychotherapy Users[a] in the Civilian U.S. Population, 1987 and 1997**

| Characteristic | Visitors to All Providers | | Visitors to Medical Doctors[b] | | Visitors to Psychologists[b] | | Visitors to Social Workers[b] | | Visitors to Other Non-M.D.'s[b,c] | |
|---|---|---|---|---|---|---|---|---|---|---|
| | 1987 | 1997 | 1987 | 1997 | 1987 | 1997 | 1987 | 1997 | 1987 | 1997 |
| | (N=993) | (N=1,136) | (n=502) | (n=756) | (n=313) | (n=379) | (n=86) | (n=135) | (n=275) | (n=169) |
| **Age (%)** | | ** | | * | | | | ** | | |
| 0-17 | 21.7 | 18.7 | 16.9 | 18.1 | 23.4 | 21.2 | 28.6 | 15.8 | 22.8 | 14.9 |
| 18-44 | 56.9 | 50.9 | 55.2 | 45.8 | 60.0 | 55.4 | 61.7 | 51.9 | 59.6 | 60.8 |
| 45-64 | 17.5 | 25.9 | 21.3 | 29.7 | 15.2 | 21.7 | 7.8 | 30.2 | 15.6 | 22.3 |
| 65+ | 3.8 | 4.5 | 6.7 | 6.4 | 1.4 | 1.8 | 1.9 | 2.1 | 2.0 | 2.0 |
| **Gender (%)** | | | | | | | | | | |
| Female | 60.1 | 59.4 | 59.8 | 59.9 | 62.9 | 60.4 | 53.2 | 64.8 | 60.9 | 64.8 |
| Male | 39.9 | 40.6 | 40.2 | 40.1 | 37.1 | 39.6 | 46.8 | 35.2 | 39.1 | 35.2 |
| **Race/ethnicity (%)** | | | | | | | | | | |
| Hispanic | 4.8 | 6.2 | 6.5 | 6.2 | 4.2 | 4.6 | 5.3 | 8.6 | 2.9 | 5.9 |
| African American, non-Hisp. | 6.0 | 6.9 | 8.6 | 7.3 | 4.4 | 5.3 | 3.9 | 1.7 | 6.0 | 9.2 |
| White, non-Hisp. | 87.3 | 85.8 | 83.1 | 85.9 | 89.9 | 88.7 | 86.4 | 89.8 | 87.9 | 83.4 |
| Other, non-Hisp. | 1.9 | 1.1 | 1.8 | 0.6 | 1.5 | 1.4 | 4.5 | 0.0 | 3.2 | 1.5 |
| **Marital status (%)** | | | | | | | | | | |
| Married | 47.9 | 45.2 | 45.5 | 47.3 | 47.8 | 43.1 | 47.3 | 43.3 | 47.4 | 36.8 |
| Single/Separ./Div./Widowed | 52.1 | 54.9 | 54.5 | 52.7 | 52.2 | 56.9 | 52.7 | 56.7 | 52.6 | 63.2 |
| **Health insurance (%)[d]** | | * | | | | *** | | | | |
| Private | 77.7 | 70.5 | 73.1 | 68.2 | 86.4 | 71.5 | 81.9 | 74.9 | 71.4 | 64.1 |
| Public only | 15.0 | 21.0 | 20.2 | 25.0 | 9.7 | 18.1 | 11.2 | 16.2 | 18.3 | 26.6 |
| None | 7.3 | 8.6 | 6.8 | 6.8 | 3.9 | 10.5 | 6.9 | 8.9 | 10.4 | 9.3 |
| **Family income (%)[e]** | | | | | | * | | | | |
| Poor to low income | 32.0 | 33.7 | 36.6 | 38.3 | 23.1 | 31.5 | 26.0 | 30.9 | 41.5 | 37.2 |
| Middle to high income | 68.0 | 66.4 | 63.4 | 61.7 | 76.9 | 68.5 | 74.0 | 69.1 | 58.5 | 62.8 |

Note. Figures are national estimates based on weighted data from the 1987 National Medical Expenditures Survey (NMES) and the 1997 Medical Expenditure Panel Survey (MEPS). SUDAAN software was used to account for the complex survey design. Year effects in this table are tested with c2 analysis (df = number of categories of the demographic characteristic - 1). Significant year effects are boxed.

[a]Psychotherapy users were those who made at least 1 visit to a provider in an office-based practice or a hospital outpatient unit where "psychotherapy/mental health counseling" was the main reason for the visit (NMES) or where "psychotherapy/counseling" was among the services received (MEPS). [b]Columns labeled with particular provider types are not mutually exclusive, as a portion of psychotherapy users (16.4% in 1987 and 23.6% in 1997) saw more than 1 provider type. [c]The most commonly given titles included: "therapist," "counselor," "mental health counselor," "occupational therapist," "physical therapist," and "nurse/nurse practitioner." [d]Private = any private insurance coverage during the year; Public only = any public insurance coverage during the year (no private coverage all year); None = no private or public coverage throughout the year. [e]Poor to low income = Below poverty line to less than 200% of poverty line; Middle to high income = 200% or more above poverty line.

*P < .05. **P < .01. ***P < .001. ****P < .0001.

**TABLE 4.**
**Average Proportion of Psychotherapy[a] Expenditures Paid Out of Pocket and by Private and Public Insurance Sources, 1987 and 1997**

| Payment source | All Visits | | Visitors to Medical Doctors | | Visitors to Psychologists | | Visitors to Social Workers | | Visitors to Other Non-M.D.'s | |
|---|---|---|---|---|---|---|---|---|---|---|
| | 1987 (*N*=10,112) | 1997 (*N*=10,010) | 1987 (*n*=3,730) | 1997 (*n*=4,541) | 1987 (*n*=2,964) | 1997 (*n*=2,865) | 1987 (*n*=676) | 1997 (*n*=1,166) | 1987 (*n*=2,742) | 1997 (*n*=1,438) |
| Out of pocket (%) | 50.9 | 37.4**** | 47.0 | 33.9**** | 53.5 | 39.4*** | 52.5 | 39.8 | 53.1 | 40.1* |
| Private insurance (%) | 28.5 | 35.1** | 24.9 | 34.0*** | 31.9 | 38.1 | 28.2 | 35.6 | 27.1 | 27.2 |
| Public insurance (%) | 19.7 | 27.6*** | 26.5 | 32.1 | 14.4 | 22.5* | 19.3 | 24.6 | 18.3 | 32.7** |

*Note.* Figures are national estimates based on weighted data from the 1987 National Medical Expenditures Survey (NMES) and the 1997 Medical Expenditure Panel Survey (MEPS). SUDAAN software was used to account for the complex survey design. Year effects in this table are tested with $c^2$ analysis ($df = 1$). Some columns do not sum to 100% because of rounding error.

[a]Psychotherapy users were those who made at least 1 visit to a provider in an office-based practice or a hospital outpatient unit where "psychotherapy/mental health counseling" was the main reason for the visit (NMES) or where "psychotherapy/counseling" was among the services received (MEPS). [b]The most commonly given titles included "therapist," "counsellor," "mental health counsellor," "occupational therapist," "counselor," "mental health counselor," "occupational therapist," "physical therapist", "physical therapist," and "nurse/nurse practitioner." [c] Proportion paid by self or family.

*$P < .05$. **$P < .01$. ***$P < .001$. ****$P < .0001$.

provider types. Across years, the vast majority (86%) of users were non-Hispanic Whites, and about two-thirds of users were middle to high income. However, the average user in 1997 was somewhat older, with this trend most pronounced among people who saw medical doctors and social workers. In 1997, psychotherapy users had more public and less private health insurance coverage, which was reflected sharply among those who saw psychologists. Psychologists were also the only provider group to be seeing a increased percentage of lower-income clients in 1997.

### Payment Sources for Psychotherapy Visits

Out-of-pocket payments for psychotherapy decreased between 1987 and 1997, with the mean proportion dropping from 51% in 1987 to 37% in 1997 (**see Table 4**). The proportion paid by private insurance sources went from 29% to 35%, and the public insurance share rose from 20% to 28%. Medical doctors were the only provider type whose psychotherapy services received a reliably higher proportion of private insurance payments in 1997. Services by psychologists and other non-M.D. providers showed the most robust increase in proportion of payments made by public insurance sources.

### References (for the Appendix)

Agency for Healthcare Research and Quality (Jan. 2001). Content Summary of the Household Interview. AHRQ Publication No. 01-P006. Rockville, MD. http://www.meps.ahrq.gov./factsheets/fs_summhcintv.htm

Agency for Healthcare Research and Quality (Feb. 2001). MEPS Fact Sheet. Rockville, MD. http://www.meps.ahrq.gov/whatismeps/bulletin.htm

Cohen, S., DiGaetano, R., and Waksberg, J. (1991). Sample Design of the 1987 Household Survey. National Medical Expenditure Survey Methods 3. Agency for Health Care Policy and Research, Publication No. 91-0037. Rockville, MD: Public Health Service.

Edwards, W. and Berlin, M. (1989, September). Questionnaires and data collection methods for the Household Survey and the Survey of American Indians and Alaska Natives (DHHS Publication No. PHS-89-3450). National Medical Expenditure Survey Methods 2, National Center for Health Services Research and Health Care Technology Assessment. Rockville, MD: Public Health Service.

## Social and Community Therapies in an Era of Deinstitutionalization

**Carole A. Anderson, Ph.D., R.N., F.A.A.N., Ohio State University**

Many of us were excited by the notion of deinstitutionalization in the 1960s. The figures show what happened. In 1955, there were 559,000 inpatients out of a population of 165 million, or 339/100,000. Comparable figures in 1998 were 51,151 patients in a population of 175 million, or 21 in 100,000. In most states many hospitals have closed and state funding has shifted to local mental health boards, which led to some integrated services and efficiencies, but a new generation of patients who are young, not passive, deny their illness, frequently have co-morbidity with drug and/or alcohol abuse, and, too often, find their way into the criminal justice system.

In 1984, Talbot and Lamb described what is needed to replace long term care: "The experience with deinstitutionalization has made clear that a comprehensive and integrated system of care for the chronically and severely mentally ill, with designated responsibility, accountability and adequate financial resources, needs to be established in the community." (Lamb, H.R., 1984)

The answer to whether that vision has been realized is "yes and no," yes because some strong community systems have been built, but no because few, if any, are both comprehensive and integrated. And all public systems are now under considerable strain, with demands and expectations increasing. The size of the homeless population, where a large percentage is mentally ill, illustrates the unmet needs and demonstrates something has gone wrong. Everywhere funding is diminishing. The result is a system stretched too thin, with holes in it and diminishing resources to support it. Importantly, this system lacks the ability to recruit and retain trained professionals.

What is needed to correct the problems is assertive community treatment including supportive teams, multiple integrated services, viable living arrangements, meaningful work, access to primary care—this population has a lot of unmet medical needs—some self management and family support, because we forget what a horrible burden it is for families of the seriously mentally ill.

But above all what is needed is well-trained professionals, making use of evidence-based practice, working in teams, and collaborating with patients and families, and with policy makers because they provide funding and making full utilization of all health professions.

That includes nursing. In our discussions, no one had mentioned school nurses, public health nurses who go into peoples homes, or pediatric nurse practitioners. The word nurse has not been mentioned. Psychiatric nursing has been around since mid-50s, contents have been part of basic nursing education since 1955, when graduate education also began. Yet nurses are often neglected in the discourse about psychiatry and mental health. The nursing profession is like mothers, valuable in its absence. When nurses are present, they are taken for granted, treated as if they are invisible. In mental health systems, the only viable roles for nurses are in inpatient settings, which is ironic because needs are so great throughout the mental health system and the skill set of nurses is so appropriate.

As a result, there has been significant decline in number of graduate programs for psychiatric nursing and numbers of students enrolled. In 2000 there were 17 fewer programs than the year before. Also, in 2000, only 413 students, or 2.2% of students, were enrolled in these programs. The existing cohort of psychiatric nurses is aging and leaving the field, and these nurses are not being replaced through training programs.

A number of steps are needed to correct these situations. Although other health professionals are mentioned, a lot of the discourse makes it seem that psychiatrists do all the front line work. I'm not sure people are convinced that isn't the case, even though we know it is not true. Policy work is needed to advocate for equal treatment legislation. Nurses need new roles to vitalize the mental health system. It is important to use all professionals and to ensure that training of those professionals is at an appropriate level and that they are doing what they have been trained to do. We also need to focus on unmet needs and bring an awareness of those needs to the public. But most of all, we need well-trained professionals.

## New Models for Treating a Dual Diagnosis

**Laura F. McNicholas, M.D., Ph.D.,**
**University of Pennsylvania**

The term dual diagnosis is a misnomer. Most of our patients have one or more substance abuse problems, plus one or more psychiatric disorders, plus medical disorders that need something done about them. When talking about dual diagnosis, what I hear from medical students is that most people have one or the other, not both. Well they do. Both ECA and the National Comorbidity Study looked at dual diagnosis and found it somewhere in the 50% range.

The issue that then comes up is which led to which and there are risk factors in both. The presence of another primary psychiatric disorder modifies the course of an addictive disorder. Usually it makes it worse. Psychiatric symptoms may develop in the course of chronic intoxication. The relation between depression and alcoholism is common. Patients who may or may not have been depressed when they started drinking frequently end up depressed with an independent diagnosis of depressive disorder. There are also psychiatric symptoms that may emerge with chronic use of a drug. Certainly with cocaine we always see it.

For patients, the symptoms become linked over time and that's also true for providers, so they don't distinguish between what is a primary psychiatric disorder and what is a substance abuse disorder. Caregivers frequently forget disorders can present at different times, and it is often difficult to distinguish between the primary and secondary disorder. Primary disorders follow patterns of normal psychiatric disorder. Secondary disorders, which we almost invariably deal with in a substance abuse population, remit when abstinence occurs.

This is especially true with depressed patients. Between 60-90% present with signs of depression, but data that suggests between 30-70% of these are secondary: diagnosis of depression and symptoms will remit when the patient becomes abstinent. But there are also patients where depression is a clear primary diagnosis. We are always dealing with primary or secondary diagnosis and the issue of appropriate treatment. We also have co-occurring problems where both the substance abuse disorder and the primary mental disorder occur at the same time.

Primary patterns of dual disorders includes high psychiatric severity

## PREVALENCE OF DUAL DISORDERS: NATIONAL STUDIES

**ECA Survey (Robins & Regeir):**

- 37% with alcohol and 53% with drug use disorder had lifetime mental d/o
- 29% with mental d/o had lifetime SUD

**Nat'l Comorbidity Study: (Kessler et al)**

- 41-66% with SUD have mental disorder
- 51% with a mental disorder have SUD
- 25-35% with SMI have had a SUD over the past 6 months
- Psychiatric inpatients & outpatients: 20-50% with concurrent SUD
- SUDs are more common among young, male, single, and less educated clients

— *Drake & Mueser; Rosenthal & Westreich*

and high substance abuse severity. The most complicated of these are schizophrenic patients who are abusing cocaine. You also can have high, moderate, or low substance abuse with high psychiatric severity, and that alters over time. High psychiatric severity patients can go, infrequently, from high or frequent level of substance abuse and to a low level, or stop.

A thorough assessment takes time and effort. A thorough history, along with the patterns and types of drugs used, is essential for both medications as well as non-therapeutic purposes, as well as understanding of the temporal relationship between drug use and psychiatric signs and symptoms. Information is gathered through interviews, standardized instruments, questionnaires, and laboratory tests. It is essential to understand the attitudes and biases of students and how they will receive information. Problems in gathering this information include denial and deception by patients who are sensitive about how they are perceived, also limited information and inadequate evaluations.

The three basic approaches to treatment are sequential—treat one and then the other—and parallel—you do one I'll do the other. But the only one that really works is the integrated model. You have to treat both at the same time and in the same system of treatment. The focus of the treatment depends on current symptoms and problems, so there is not necessarily a 50-50 balance. The approach to treatment is to manage what is going on with the patient. The most important thing is to identify the problem.

You have to engage the person in treatment. You frequently hear "that's not what I'm here for. I'm here for my schizophrenia, not my alcohol abuse or for my depression"... hear from other direction, "my primary problem is not depression." Then you have to engage the person, educate them about treatment, and introduce the idea of recovery, frequently a foreign concept. You have to facilitate rehabilitation and facilitate self-help groups and educate about appropriate therapy. Some won't take medication for substance use though there is medication for variety of them, just as some don't want to take appropriate pharmacotherapy for psychiatric problems.

Collaboration with case managers is essential. A lot of patients need more intensive management that most physicians can give on their schedules. You need to figure out appropriate hospital services, appropriate outpatient services, appropriate pharmacotherapy, and appropriate social services. Inpatient hospitalization is used for stabilization when necessary, though this is frequently difficult in managed care situations. Partial hospital and intensive outpatient care can be very useful managing dual diagnosis patients, as can supportive housing and community residential programs. If you have patients living on the street or under a bridge, you are not going to get very far with them. You need to know community resources for counseling and supportive care and be sure to use appropriate services.

Case managers provide patients with a single point of contact. The best case managers are masters level psychiatric nurses who understand pharmacology and both the aspects of psychiatric and substance abuse disorders and the systems the patient needs to access. That single point of contact is essential for the engagement and retention of the patient. The case manager does the coordination, planning, and monitoring, works with the physician, advocates for the patient and provides liaison with the community. The approach decreases fragmentation of patient care for somebody knows what is going on with the patient at all levels and provides links to care.

In this era of "cost effectiveness" and "treatment efficacy," clinicians need to think differently about what they do and how they do it. Physicians can't do what they did 15 years ago and expect it to work or to get paid for it. The number of inpatient days has been reduced —more is not better—with more focus on partial programs and outpatient programs and services. A lot of patients we see are moderate and moderate patients can be helped. The ones that block up the system are the persistently mentally ill with severe substance abuse disorder and that's who we really need to talk about in intensive outpatient care and case management.

There is not one program that will work in every system, so you need to know what will work best for you and how to access that program. You need a full continuum of care for patients, including manualized therapies, for these patients can respond as well as other patients. Frequently we don't think of that because we think they won't respond to supportive therapy, but they do. You can effectively integrate treatment and maximize control of both psychiatric and substance abuse disorders but you can't cure either one of them. They are chronic relapsing disorders: there are going to be slips, there are going to be relapses. The issue is to make the slips and relapses manageable and least uncomfortable for the patient in an effective fashion.

## Discussion Highlights, Session II

### Psychopharmacology & Psychotherapy

— Psychotherapy is not a universal solvent: It doesn't work for all disorders and not all psychotherapies work. Psychotherapeutic approaches are probably most successful with problems that affect learning, memory and behavior, and also may help reduce environmental risk factors and delay the onset of illness. Efficacy for most of the evidence-based therapies, as outlined in manuals, has been established in at least two clinical trials, meeting the same Food and Drug Administration requirements for new drugs. Not all psychotherapies have met these rigorous criteria. Criticisms of manualized treatment as "cookbook" therapy that doesn't consider individual patient needs often comes from practitioners who either haven't learned any of these approaches or are personally invested in other approaches.

### Evidence-Based Psychotherapy

— Some psychologists complain that manualized therapies are boring, that they went into the field to learn about individuals, and that the use of these cookbook approaches reduces then to being mere technicians. That complaint suggests the question of professional satisfaction needs to be addressed.

— What is currently done under the guise of psychotherapy by both medical and non-medical people is variable. What is important is that they learn to listen to patients and to understand them. Once they master this, learning another strategy— one that is time-limited and can help with specific problems— is relatively easy. Since most people can't afford extensive therapy, both approaches are needed. Currently, too many patients only get once-a-month or once-in-a-crisis sessions, with results that too often are not very good. Accordingly, therapists need to be taught how to listen as well as how to treat in a way that produces concrete and measurable results. Until that happens, the translation of evidence-based approaches into real world practice is not going to occur.

— What is needed is a good systematic and updated review of the effectiveness of different psychotherapies for all disorders, not conducted by practitioners in the field. The same kind of review is needed for residency and graduate training programs in psychiatry, psychology, and social work to determine their relevance to current practice and exposure of trainees to evidence-based therapies. One way to do this would be to bring together those who make decisions about training programs. Residency and graduate training programs for non-mental health professions also should be expanded to include material on patient evaluation, psychotropic medicine and indications for referral.

## Training of MD's

— The challenge of training residents and implementing evidence-based therapies is compounded by the fact that many training programs rely exclusively on part-time faculty members, many of whom are in mid to late career and have no experience with these different therapies and a commitment to their own "one type fits all" approach. In part this is a guild issue, but it also involves the broader question of who provides care and who needs training; and it includes psychologists and psychiatric social workers, not just psychiatrists. Indeed, because of reimbursement rates, increasingly psychiatrists are not the professionals providing therapy, which increases the importance of appropriate training for the entire array of mental health professionals.

## Changing Roles

— The role of psychiatrists in providing mental health care is changing. More are getting away from working directly with patients and, instead, are now supervising care and working with psychiatric social workers and others who do the actual therapy, perhaps taking on only the more complicated cases. Accordingly, psychiatry students need to be taught to evaluate the skills and competencies of those with whom they will work.

## Teaching of Non MD's

— Mental health professions confront the challenge of finding ways to teach students the way that they will practice. Training for these professions tends to be separate though practice is usually both multidisciplinary and multi-professional. Mental health professionals also have the responsibility for training non-mental health professionals to recognize and treat mental illness. The fact that psychiatry is listed in the "other" category indicates how far psychiatry is from mainstream medicine and how difficult it is for psychiatry to provide this needed training.

— The involvement of social workers in psychotherapy has increased over past decades, though as a group they are poorly informed about different therapies and don't know about existing guidelines. When informed, they tend to find the guidelines "interesting," but prefer to follow expert opinion and consensus about what works, rather than relying on scientific evidence.

## Community Approaches

— Closer collaboration is needed between those who do research and those in practice, but this will be difficult to achieve. Those in community-based programs complain that research is not relevant to what they do, while researchers say they need to stay separate from practice and that if they have to pass a relevancy test they will lose the ability to generate new knowledge. Even so, research needs to be more responsive to questions from the field and, when appropriate, lead practitioners to answers that are already there.

## Advances in Therapies

— As a discipline, psychiatry is staying constant in numbers but with increasing expectations and many new roles. In addition to traditional roles and trying to integrate new science, psychiatry has taken on increasingly different roles that are not part of traditional analysis, of prevention, genetic studies, systems leadership, accountable and rigorous diagnosis and treatment. The field also is responding to the critique that biological psychiatry has led to a dimunition of humanistic psychiatry, that people have forgotten to listen and work with the patient as  person.

## Evidence-Based Rx

— Problems within the discipline could be corrected by using and understanding quality evidence. Applying evidence across the board would make an important cultural change. Along with primary care, psychiatry feels discriminated against and treated as second class by others in the medical profession. Communications teaching must be competency-based and persistent in the curriculum. More explicit expectations of the outcomes of a psychiatry clerkship would improve the value of psychiatry as an intrinsic part of medical education.

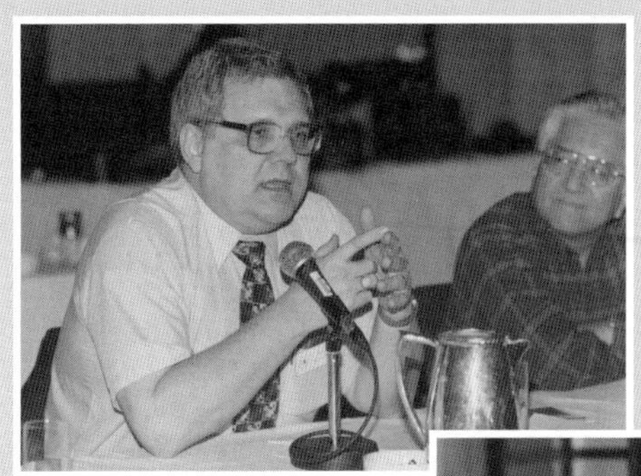

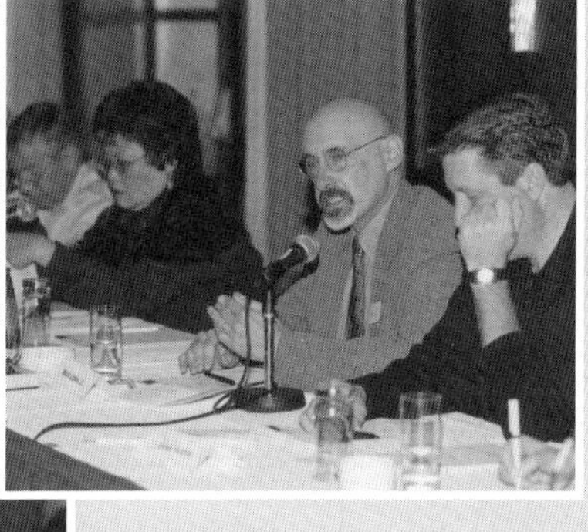

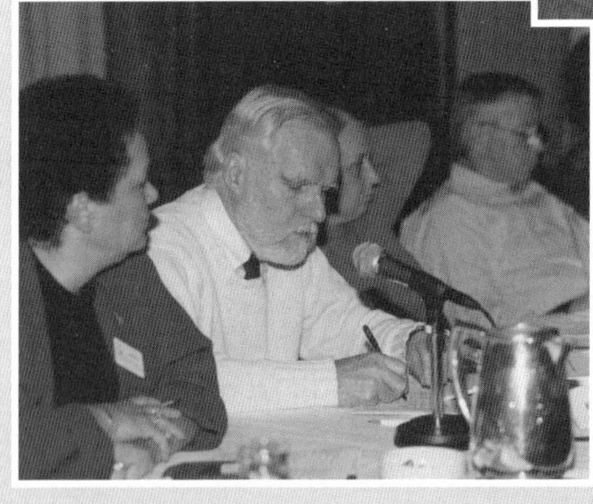

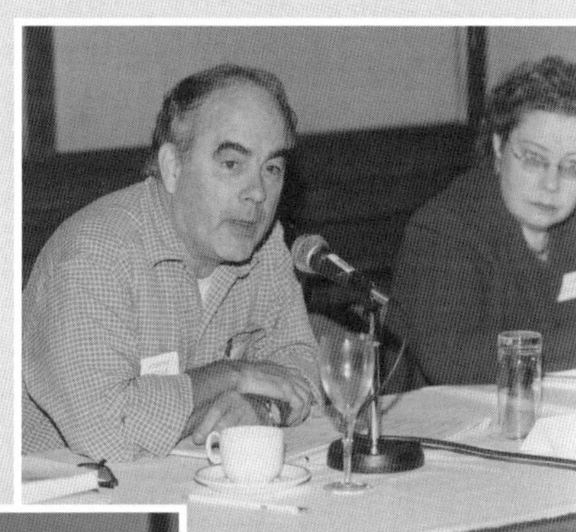

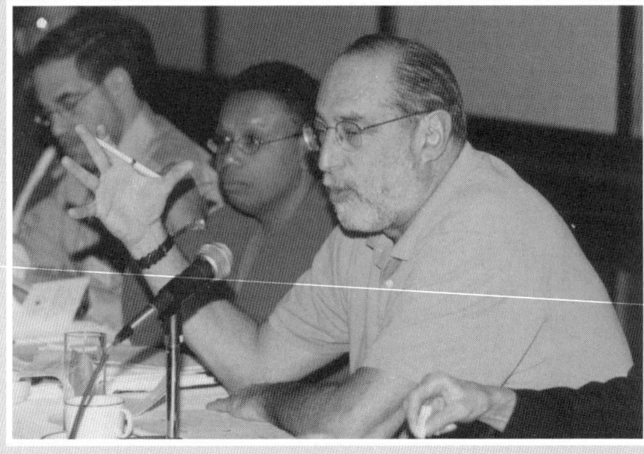

# Session III

## Care of Children, Adolescents and the Elderly: Prevention and Treatment Issues

*Historically, these populations have lagged far behind the adult mentally ill in provision of effective, accessible therapy and clinical research into their disorders. At the same time, the child and adolescent mental health needs are urgent. In this session the current state of the rather sparse field of child psychiatry is presented. Important and increasing roles for additional professionals in preventing and treating child mental disorders is elaborated, specifically, the education and training for pediatricians and professionals engaged in school-based mental health. Also, the exciting developments of the emergent field of Geriatric Psychiatry and its related education and training issues are provided.*

# 21st Century School Mental Health Providers: Trends in Education, Standards and Practice

**By Kevin P. Dwyer, MA, NCSP**

**Abstract:**

This article examines the positive trends in the preparation and practices of three mental health professions serving in our nation's schools: school counselors, school psychologists and school social workers. These three professions are addressing some of the mental health and behavioral needs of our Nation's children through prevention, early intervention, targeted, and intensive interventions. This article will discuss these professions' educational requirements for credentialing, their numbers and movement toward a systemic comprehensive mental health delivery system. One of these professions, school psychology, will be addressed in greater depth. Barriers to establishing a public mental health cadre in the schools are addressed. Partnerships in pre-service preparation and practice are explored in the recommendations.

## Background

Over the past quarter century, child rearing has become far more complex and frequently less supportive of children's mental health (National Research Council, Institute of Medicine, 2000). Compounding this negative change in family and community supports for mental wellness are the recent tragic terrorist violence and school shootings, leaving children and families feeling more vulnerable and anxious.

In a report by the National Research Council, Institute of Medicine, (1999) the changed structure of the family including higher parental employment, longer work-days, and high divorce rates, resulted in more children in the care of others, or on their own. The U.S. Department of Health and Human Services (1996) reported that children in child care rose from 30% in 1970 to 70% in 1993. Child poverty rates also increased during those years to an alarming 22% in the late 1980's (Children's Defense Fund, 1996). Complex factors can negatively affect normal child development (Felson, 1996). Combinations of environmental risk factors such as exposure to violence, poverty, poor prenatal and neonatal care and adverse experiences at home, in the community and school, "...especially those that are longstanding...seem likely to induce a mental disorder in all but the hardiest of children." (Page 129, U.S. Department of Health and Human Services, 1999). Post-traumatic stress disorder related to experiencing violence or tragedy has a marked impact on the motivation, attention and learning of affected children (Hess & Copeland, 1997).

During the early half of the 1990's almost all risk factors peaked among children (U.S. Department of Health & Human Services, 1996). Homicide and suicide rates were at their highest. Fighting in school and class disruptions were endemic. Weapons in school and adolescent substance abuse were at record levels. In one study, reports of psychosocial or mental health problem pediatric office visits, increased from 7% in 1979 to 18.7% in 1996 (Kelleher, *et al.*, 1999). Similarly the Surgeon General's report noted that 21% of children and adolescents ages 9 to 17 had a diagnosable mental or addictive disorder associated with at least minimum functional impairment (Page 123, U.S. Department of Health and Human Services, 1999). These factors, combined with the added stress of terrorist attacks, have resulted in the realization that universal early childhood and school mental health programs must become a national priority.

Economic and social changes in the past quarter century have also placed greater pressures on schools for what some may see as competing goals. Business demands highly literate, technologically and math skilled graduates for its workforce. Federal and state policymakers have echoed this demand in formulating higher standards and accountability measures for defining good schools, academic success, and graduation requirements. Leaders had been less supportive for meeting the heightened health and mental health needs of children. Yet, during these years advances in behavioral science and neuroscience clarified the links between mental health status and academic achievement (National Research Council and Institute of Medicine, 2000).

The fundamental mission of the schools in preparing young persons to function effectively as workers, parents, and citizens is enduring. However, today schools need the infrastructure and mental health providers in place to support the fundamental unmet needs in the mental health field. Mental wellness supports the achievement and behavioral mission of schools. This needed infrastructure goes far beyond teachers. Teachers can become partners in promoting mental health but cannot and should not be expected to have the knowledge, skills or responsibilities of school or child psychologists or social workers. The infrastructure requires easy access by teachers to consultation and training to establish caring school environments that promote mental health.

To address these child mental health needs, Surgeon General Satcher developed a "national action agenda for children's mental health" (U.S. Department of Health and Human Services, 2000). This report stressed the importance of prevention and the role of schools in developmental learning for the promotion of mental health. The overreaching vision of that report states:

> Mental health is a critical component of children's learning and general health. Fostering social and emotional health in children as a part of healthy child development must therefore be a national priority. Both the promotion of mental health in children and the treatment of mental disorders should be major public health goals. To achieve these goals, the *Surgeon General's National Action Agenda for Children's Mental Health* takes its guiding principles and commitment to:
>
> 1. Promoting the recognition of mental health as an essential part of child health;
> 2. Integrating family, child and youth-centered mental health services into all systems that serve children and youth;
> 3. Engaging families and incorporating the perspectives of children and youth in the development of all mental healthcare planning;
> 4. Developing and enhancing a public-private health infrastructure to support these efforts to the fullest extent possible. (p. 3)

**New Directions**

A century ago infectious diseases placed students at risk and public health measures entered the policies and practices of schools. Today immunizations are required for school entry, vision and hearing screening are common, and school environments are required to be designed and inspected to be free of toxins and environmental hazards. Whole communities have laws and policies to address public health and safety. Yesterday's problems have been replaced by a new set of problems related to behavior. Fire drills have been replaced by crisis plans to address a multitude of once unbelievable scenarios. Public health efforts of inoculating children with behavioral skills, building on resilience and removing environmental behavioral toxins have become efforts worthy of community support.

A quarter century of data are unequivocal: with proper training and infrastructure support, many children can be prevented from becoming children with emotional and behavioral disorders (Ysseldyke, 1984; Albee & Gullotta, 1997). When children at risk are taught the fundamental skills of behavior, social communication and problem solving they are less likely to be determined disabled and in need of special education and related services (Knoff & Batsche, 1995). Research has also informed us that early interventions are almost always more effective than late interventions for children at-risk or those beginning to fail to function successfully (Walker, 1999; Walker & Rankin, 1983).

During that same quarter century child-related professions were beginning to recognize their obligation to learn and apply proven practices to improve systems of care for children in this more stressful and less psychologically supportive social environment. Childcare program standards were developed and Head Start was expanded. Manuals of proven prevention, early and targeted interventions and intensive interventions were produced and widely disseminated. Proposals were made to plan comprehensive, coordinated systems of prevention and care for children's mental well-being (National Research Council and Institute of Medicine, 2001; Dwyer & Osher, 2000; Center for Mental Health Services, July, 1999; Greenberg, *et al.*, 2001; Albee & Gullotta, 1997).

The negative impact of toxic social changes moved many to recommend restructuring service systems toward universal primary prevention and toward effectively addressing risk factors. Public health reaches its prevention goals by providing a strategic, planned approach to health, mental health and education practices and services. According to Hamburg (1998) the essential features of the public health model include:

a. Community collaborative, multidisciplinary problem identification and community focused, universal solutions.

b. Monitoring of health (including mental health) data to establish the magnitude and nature of the problem and track trends and related risk factors.

c. Analyzing of data on risk and related factors.

d. Designing and implementing interventions and their evaluation.

e. Providing community wide outreach, education and information as to what works (moving to scale).

The professional changes detailed in this article build on the public health model adapted for the school setting (Adelman, 1996; Dryfoos, 1994; Dwyer & Osher, 2000; Hamburg, 1998; Knoff, 1996; Institute of Medicine, 1997; Walker 1999). Its implementation through training, policy and practice is beginning to be realized. For example, the Policy Leadership Cadre for Mental Health in Schools (Adelman, 2001), gaining consensus from a wide array of constituents has developed resource guidelines for this public *mental* health agenda. Furthermore, new directions in graduate training enable the desired outcomes of mental health promotion for all children, targeted early intervention for those at risk and, intensive intervention for those children with mental, emotional and behavioral problems.

Figure 1. provides the theoretical structure that schools are beginning to use to ensure that all children are supported in negotiating

**FIGURE 1**
**Expanded Public Health School Service Model**

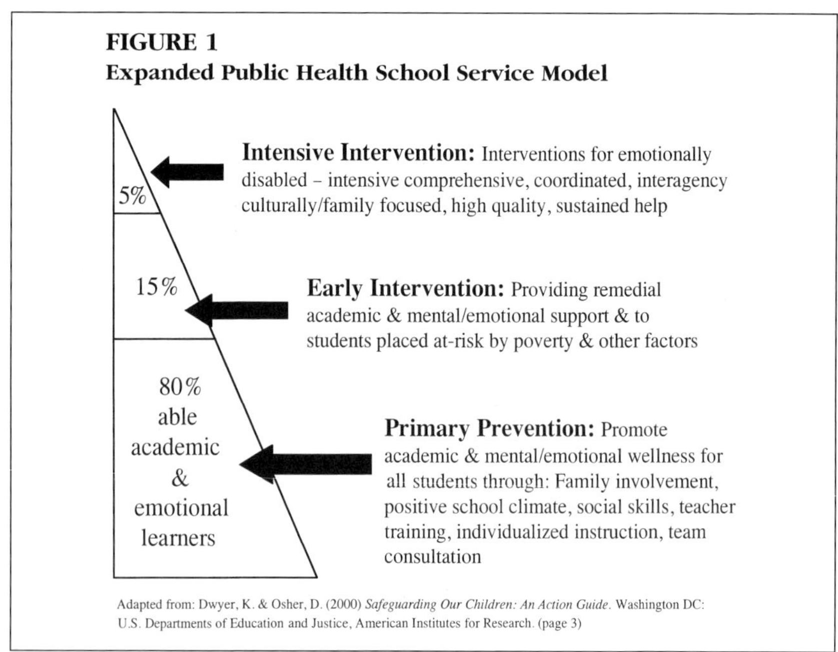


Adapted from: Dwyer, K. & Osher, D. (2000) *Safeguarding Our Children: An Action Guide*. Washington DC: U.S. Departments of Education and Justice, American Institutes for Research. (page 3)

the developmental processes of achieving appropriate academic and social skills (Adelman & Taylor, 1999; Learning First Alliance, 2001). This model requires planned integration of community-based, school-wide prevention-intervention services, aligned to allow inclusion, transition and generalization of fundamental building blocks of social-emotional learning (Curtis & Stollar, 1995; Elias & Tobias, 1996). The model also requires complete coordinated planning between school and community mental health providers with schools being the center for service delivery. Such planned integrated mental health and school health clinics have been shown to be effective in reducing behavior problems and increasing academic achievement (Lodge, 1998).

Recognizing this need for promoting mentally healthy environments and for implementing targeted interventions for those at risk and ensuring effective intensive interventions for severe mental disorders in school communities requires major changes in the training, preparation and support by a range of mental health providers, as well as support from educators, families and other child caregivers. Three professions among the many that have changed and modified their professional training and practice standards in response to the changing needs of our nation's children and families are school counselors, school psychologists and school social workers. They are not alone in their responsiveness but this article will focus on these three professions and their roles among the mental health professions.

## School Mental Health Providers

Thirty years ago school mental health service as part of schooling was quite rare (Fagan, 1995). There was little thought about addressing the prevention of mental, emotional and behavioral problems in school. Children with serious emotional and mental health disorders were frequently educated in separate settings, if at all (Knitzer, Steinberg & Fleisch, 1990). Mental health service in schools was an afterthought. In 1975, with the passage of the federal Special Education and Related Services Law (PL94-142) for children with disabilities (including "seriously emotionally disturbed") psychological, counseling and social work services were mandated for children with disabilities who required such service to learn. Similarly, under the revisions of the Elementary and Secondary Education Act, (1986) children placed at risk by poverty were afforded counseling, psychological and social work services funded by that federal resource, at the discretion of the local school system.

Before 1975, the total number of school psychologists nationally was estimated to be about 5000, a ratio of one school psychologist for about every 9000 students (Fagan & Sachs Wise, 2000). School counselors were more common, and found in most high schools. High school counselors were traditionally academic advisors, arranging class schedules and giving guidance for college and vocational preparation. School social workers, as a distinct social work profession, were even fewer in number than school psychologists.

Although "vocational guidance counseling" in high school was common after World War II, school psychology and school social work services were rare. These professions were predominantly employed in the northeast and north-central states, primarily in urban areas, close to existing university training programs. For example, prior to 1970, about 70% of school psychologists were employed by city school systems. Many states and most of the 15,000 school districts had no such professional service (Fagan & Sachs Wise, 2000).

From its early years, counseling as a school service was integrated more fully into the certification of educators, and usually required a teaching certificate and teaching experience as preparation for counselor certification (Hollis & Wantz, 1997). Secondary school counseling education was federally supported during the "Cold War" through the National Defense Education Act, providing graduate scholarships in career counseling to help counsel youth into taking the courses needed to prepare for higher education in science. Counseling services, like school librarians, were also required for high schools to be accredited by regional accreditation boards. School counseling originally focused on guidance counseling in vocation and educational choice (Hollis & Wantz, 1997). School social work, as a distinct profession of importance, is far newer (see Manderscheid & Henderson, Eds. 1998). Over a half century ago the term "visiting teacher" was synonymous with school social worker and the profession's training standards were less rigorous.

**New Roles and Responsibilities**

School counselors, psychologists and social workers fall generically under the heading of "student or pupil service" among the education (kindergarten through 12th grade) professions. Typically hired by local school systems, they are state credentialed professionals whose responsibilities include mental and behavioral health and strategies for addressing many cognitive, physical and environmental factors related to learning and adjustment. As pupil service professionals, they frequently team with other professionals including school nurses, occupational and physical therapists and speech-language therapists, among others (National Alliance of Pupil Services Organizations, 1994).

The three professions have both distinct and overlapping school functions that reflect the interplay of children's academic learning, social competence, and mental health. For example, all three are prepared to provide counseling services to children and families concerning learning and behavior including motivation and mental health problems. All utilize consultation skills with school staff and families. All three are trained to address ecological factors such as having schools better connect with alienated families, training teachers to use positive behavioral interventions and caring to address behavior, and social skill reinforcement that build resilience in children and youth and reduce the dangers of risk factors (Elias & Tobias, 1996). Distinctions relate to training, role definition, and intensity of functions and complexity of targeted interventions among other factors. For example school psychologists may have more intensive training and supervised experience in mental health, learning and behavior problems and necessary individualized interventions, whereas counselor's training may address developmental motivation and self-esteem of learners, and school social workers focus on coordinated service management.

They all are required to provide specific *related services* to children with disabilities receiving special education services, including those children classified as *emotionally disturbed* (p. 12424, Code of Federal Regulations 34 CFR Part 300.24, March 19, 1999). These *related services* include: planning and designing individualized academic and behavioral intervention plans; parent training and counseling; transition services; and a wide array of psychological services including individual and group psychological counseling and social work services, including case management.

The three professions are listed together in federal and state documents describing the components of comprehensive school health programs (Institute of Medicine, 1997). Generically they, "...promote the mental, emotional, and social health of students and deal with problems that interfere with teaching and learning." (*ibid.*, p. 71). This spectrum includes prevention, early and intensive interventions to students, staff and families of students as well as coordinating services with community mental health providers and related agencies.

The three professions are more likely today than decades ago to participate on *school-wide improvement teams* (Learning First Alliance, 2001). School-wide improvement teams are district supported school teams responsible for implementing education reforms developed by the local education agency. School psychologists and other pupil service professions assist these teams in addressing concerns about school climate, curriculum and instruction, behavior strategies, discipline procedures, crisis planning and other educational policies and practices (Dwyer & Osher, 2000; Allensworth & Kolbe, 1987). This function of school improvement teams is critical to the implementation of the public health model in schools. These professions have been called the "coaches for mental health promotion" on these school-wide teams (Prothrow-Stith, 2001). Their inclusion enables those interested in academic reforms and school improvements to integrate psychosocial development into those plans and reduce the behavioral barriers to academic learning caused by ignoring psychosocial development. This integration of mental health and academics using the team approach is highlighted in the federal document *Safeguarding Our Children: An Action Guide* (Dwyer & Osher, 2000) among others and has been endorsed by twenty-six national mental health and education associations including the American Academy of Pediatrics, American Academy of Child and Adolescent Psychiatry, the American Psychiatric Association, the National Education Association, and National School Boards Association, among others.

Figure 2, adapted from *Safeguarding Our Children: An Action Guide* graphically displays this teaming partnership for addressing both the universal prevention issues and the individual student concerns. It displays the necessary mental health planning connection between improving the ecology of the school in addressing the academic and psychosocial needs of all, and including early interventions for those at risk, in coordination with individualized intensive interventions for those with mental and emotional problems that block learning and adjustment.

**FIGURE 2**
**School Prevention/Intervention Teams**

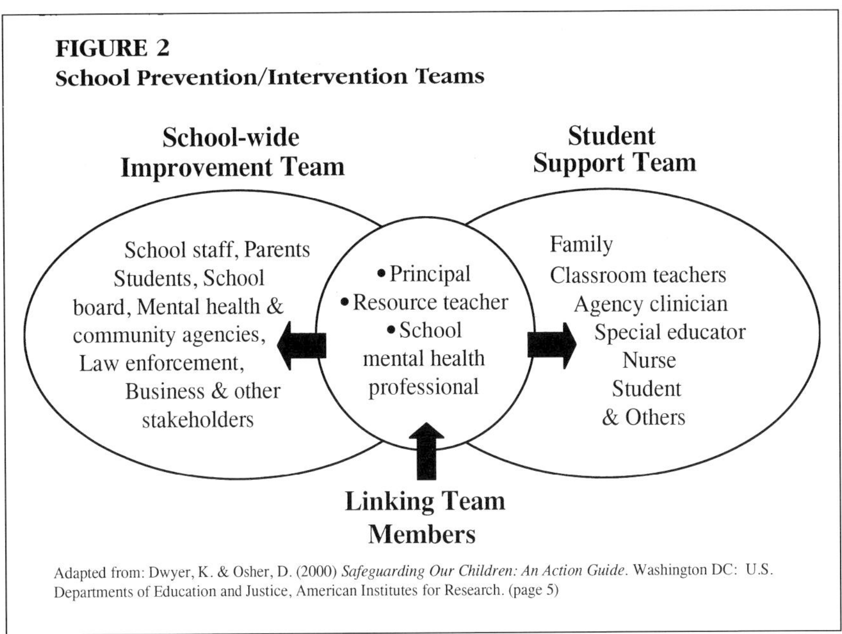


Adapted from: Dwyer, K. & Osher, D. (2000) *Safeguarding Our Children: An Action Guide.* Washington DC: U.S. Departments of Education and Justice, American Institutes for Research. (page 5)

These three professions collaborate with others (including, teacher, family, administrator, and agency providers) on school *student support teams* (see Figure 2) responsible for addressing individual student mental health, education and social welfare issues as they relate to learning and development. They, along with school nurses, serve as school links to private and public health, mental health and other agency providers in establishing collaborative service plans and agreements. They are frequently responsible for reporting detailed information about behavior and observable effects, both positive and adverse, of pharmacological and other therapeutic treatments to providers and families. They play a key role in helping children and families transition from hospitals and other settings back to school.

Student support teams are effective when they utilize school reform to address early the risk factors that lead children to manifest behavior and mental health problems. Teams that quickly plan the appropriate comprehensive services for children with serious mental health disorders increase such children's social and academic progress. Properly resourced, these teams use their skills to prevent the failed process - where children are identified with emotional or behavioral problems only after their regular classroom teachers cannot manage them or they refuse to attend school, commit a violent act or attempt suicide.

Accurate data on the deployment and the delivery of services by these three mental health professions are not readily available. However team consultation for teachers and families appears to be a common professional service. Curtis and colleagues (1999) surveyed the National Association of School Psychologist members and noted over 97% provided consultation services to teachers and families. 82% of school psychologists sampled provided some psychological counseling services to children and families, and over 70% provided teacher in-service training. Slightly more than 50% of their time was spent on this array of services, the rest being dedicated to diagnostic services. Nastasi and colleagues (1998) found that school psychologists working in 103 innovative practice school settings were significantly different from their peers in more traditional clinical settings. School psychologists emphasize a broad comprehensive approach to treatment, spending 70% or more of their time providing consultation and staff and parent training as well as management and evaluation of programs, and very little time on diagnosis for special education placement. When innovative comprehensive mental health services were provided, these programs included partnerships with clinical mental health providers (including school health clinics) and community agencies. Those exemplary programs included prevention and intervention services available to all children and families, funded from multiple sources, including Medicaid.

Among many school psychologists, the practice role had changed from screening and diagnosis to a more complete array of services including cognitive behavioral counseling, consultation, teacher/ parent training and program evaluation. This change has been slowly progressing according to several national surveys of school psychologists (Reshly & Wilson, 1989; 1992).

### Standards for the Preparation of School Counselors, Psychologists and School Social Workers

The graduate training of professional school psychologists and counselors most frequently occurs in graduate schools of education. Departments of psychology and social work also prepare professional school psychologists and school social workers. These three professions are usually credentialed (certified or licensed) by each state's department of education; however, they may also be subject to other state licensing boards. Each has a dedicated national professional association, as well as affiliation with generic professional organizations (such as the American Counseling Association, American Psychological Association, and National Association of Social Work). As professions, school counseling, school psychology and school social work each have standards for practice, standards for credentialing and codes of ethics established and promoted through their national professional associations. Each plays a role in reviewing and approving university training programs and related internship experience and settings. For example, the National Association of Social Workers has graduate training standards for entry into the social work professions of which school social work is one specialty. These standards are used by the School Social Work Association of America (Mandalwitz, 2001).Generally, each profession requires a minimum of two years of post-baccalaureate graduate school education. The minimum of a 48 graduate semester hour Masters degree program for school counseling or a minimum 60 graduate semester hour Masters/ Specialist degree program for school psychology and school social work, including supervised internship experience is required prior to applying for certification or licensure to practice in the schools. All three professions have current, updated standards for professional practice in the school community. Another paradigm shift in practice over the past quarter century includes an emphasis on measures of accountability (Reschly & Ysseldyke, 1995). All three professions train for and recommend practice outcome accountability, moving away from reliance on process requirements alone (American School Counselors Association, 1997; National Association of School Psychologists, 2000; National Association of Social Workers, 1992).

As noted above, the professions of school counseling and school psychology have standards for coursework and supervised experience required for state certification or licensure that prepare them for integrating mental health into our nation's schools. Graduate school programs are accredited for school counseling and school psychology and for school social work. Integrating education and mental health, these programs are preparing a cadre of professionals equipped to address the public health framework of developmentally appropriate universal prevention and intervention programs in our nation's schools.

## School Psychology

The National Council for Accreditation of Teacher Education (NCATE) accredits schools of education at the graduate level with the training standards of the National Association of School Psychologists (NASP) being applied to school psychology programs in those graduate schools. A candidate who graduates from a program approved by NASP and who passes the National Examination in School Psychology administered by the Educational Testing Service (Praxis II) is awarded the National Certificate in School Psychology by the National School Psychology Certification Board.

Approved graduate programs in school psychology preparing entry-level professional school psychologists for practice in schools provide *specialist-level* preparation through a three-year, full-time graduate program. These programs include a minimum of 60 graduate semester hours plus a supervised, one academic year, 1200 clock hour internship. That internship must include at least 600 hours in school settings.

School psychology candidates must demonstrate competency in eleven domains including: (1) data-based decision-making and accountability (including connecting diagnosis to effective interventions); (2) behavioral and mental health consultation and collaboration skills as well as systems consultation skills; (3) knowledge of the human learning process, effective instruction and the development of cognitive/academic skills; (4) human developmental process relating to behavioral, affective, adaptive and social skills including behavioral and cognitive interventions and counseling; (5) knowledge of student diversity in development and learning, including individual differences and the influences of biological, social, cultural, ethnic, experiential, gender and linguistic factors; (6) skills in school system organization, policies and practices; (7) prevention science, crisis and mental health interventions; (8) home/school/community collaboration, family systems, culture and public, private agency systems; (9) research and program evaluation including translating research into practice; (10) school psychology practice and development including ethical, professional, and legal standards and; (11) information technology. Expanded descriptions of these domains of training and practice can be found in the Standards for Training and Field Placement Programs in School Psychology (NASP, 2000). For example school psychology programs are expected to prepare candidates to carry out empirically proven, theory-based practice in the natural setting. They should be familiar with ecological evaluation techniques, examining not only the child, but also the school and home environmental factors and their influence on that child's functioning. Students are expected to demonstrate their skills in designing, implementing, and evaluating interventions at the individual, classroom, school and system levels.

**School Counseling**

School counseling graduates from a graduate program accredited by the Council for Accreditation of Counseling and Related Education Programs (CACREP) have a minimum of 48 semester hours of graduate study. This sequenced study includes the following curriculum areas: (1) professional identity; (2) social cultural diversity; (3) human growth and development; (4) career development; (5) helping relationships; (6) group work; (7) assessment and; (8) research and program evaluation. Along with this core, the following skills are required: current trends in school counseling and educational systems including curriculum; academic and student service programs, including strategies designed to enhance the learning environment; teaming skills and the understanding of community opportunities and barriers that impede students; technology in education and; legal and ethical issues related to school counseling. The program also requires a 600 clock hour supervised internship in a school setting.

**School Social Work**

The Council on Social Work Education accredits graduate programs in social work, of which school social work is a specialty whose standards for professional preparation were revised in 1992 (NASW, 1992.). Program preparation beyond professional social work includes knowledge and understanding of local education agencies, educational process, laws and due process. The curriculum includes: human behavior and social environment theory; nature of systematic assessment; methods of social work intervention; local education agency organization; reciprocal influences of home, school and community; a wide array of interventions and their evaluation as well as interpreting social work to administrators and policy makers. Standards for school social work practice include: applying NASW's professional ethics; collaborative teamwork to overcome institutional barriers and service gaps; prevention in-service training for school staff; data maintenance and utilization; identifying children in need of services; using objective measures of behavior, social skills and attitudes, and developing intervention plans; providing consultation; providing culturally competent interventions; providing strength focused and empowering services; providing connections to community resources; respecting confidentiality; using mediation and conflict resolution in problem resolution; and advocating for children and families.

**Access to Services**

Today, after significant changes in graduate preparation and state certification standards these three school professions now constitute the largest cadre of "...primary providers of mental health services for children." (p. 172. Department of Health and Human Services, 1999). As a group, in collaboration with other school staff, they provide between 70-80% of the mental health services to this nation's children with mental illness (Burns, *et al.* 1995).

However, in too many school systems their services remain limited in scope to eligibility diagnosis for special education, course scheduling and vocational preparation. Attention to both prevention and treatment remain limited. Although school mental health provides a significant service, direct and consultative intervention services continue to reach only a small number of children with serious mental health problems. The U.S. Surgeon General's comprehensive report on mental health (Department of Health and Human Services, 1999) confirmed that these school mental health services, in combination with other clinical services, continue to reach only a small percentage of the 3-5% of children with serious emotional disturbance who need services.

Adelman & Taylor (1999) indicate that school-based service delivery is not responding to the needs of children, or reaching pre-service training and professional association practice standards. The known neglect of children's mental health by the nation's systems of care continues. It has been shown that schools are not addressing problems early. Surveys have shown schools did not address appropriately problems already recognized by parents at age 3 until the children had been exposed to a long series of failed, superficial interventions (Forness, 2001). Dr. Forness, using research evidence, appeals for a system of early intervention, teacher training and team screening, "for emotional and behavioral disorders early in the school years, just as they are screened for visual acuity and other health problems." (*ibid.* p. 21).

The Surgeon General noted the ongoing neglect in that fewer than 30% of children with disabling mental health problems receive needed services through any system and only one-in-five needing intensive service receive services from a clinical professional such as a psychiatrist. Furthermore, many more children are at risk of experiencing such problems (Department of Health and Human Services, 1999).

School mental health promotion and prevention programs are yet to be studied as to their availability for school age children. Although more schools than ever are applying psycho-social skill development programs, prevention research is not being implemented in a systematic manner that enables us to determine if there has been any measurable impact on this epidemic of mental emotional and behavioral problems (Adelman, 2001). No one knows how many of the 91,000 public schools have exemplary, coordinated mental health promotion programs in place or if those programs are evaluated.

Some efforts are in place. Professionals have been trained and effective programs have been developed, researched and implemented in school communities (Nastasi, *et al.*, 1998). Over the past quarter century, many innovations have demonstrated that effective services can be provided, that resources can be redeployed and that children's mental wellness can be improved (Greenberg, Domitrovich & Baumberger, 2001). Some of these innovations include evidence-based school-wide prevention and skill development programs, such as the Bully Prevention Program (Elliott, 1998), the Social Awareness-Social Problem Solving Project (Elias & Tobias, 1996) and Project ACHIEVE (Knoff & Batsche, 1995). Early intervention programs for children placed at risk by poverty, community decay, violence and drug addictions have also been replicated in the schools (Kazdin, 1991). Promoting Alternative/Thinking Strategies (Greenberg, *et al.*, 1998) and I Can Problem Solve (Shure, 1997) are two social skill programs that have been shown to reduce aggressive behavior in schools and symptoms of anxiety and depression. The Iowa Strengthening Families Program (Kumpher, *et al.*, 1988) provides parents and their children training and support, reducing conduct disorder and substance abuse problems (USDHHS, 2001). Multisystemic Therapy (Henggler, 1996) functional family therapy, cognitive behavioral therapies, wraparound services and other effective intensive clinical services, as well as improvements in special and regular education and family advocacy, have produced encouraging results (USDHHS, 1999; Adelman & Taylor, 2000).

The comprehensive intervention model described here (see Figure 1) utilizes combinations of these evidence-based practices in a planned, developmentally appropriate integrated program where services are aligned to ensure the development of effective coping and problem solving skills. Thus a child who is receiving an evidence-based treatment for a specific fear or phobia can have that treatment reinforced by school staff within the classroom and other natural environments. Durable treatments, according to Weisz (Department of Health & Human Services, 2001) are applied with fidelity to a structured, manualized plan. Schools are an excellent environment for implementing such treatments for the most troubling and prevalent child and adolescent disorders— anxiety, depression, behavioral and attention-deficit hyperactivity disorder— among others.

Although many effective, proven interventions are being piloted in schools, none of these movements have yet been brought to scale to improve the mental wellness of significant numbers of our nation's children. According to Weisz, "These beneficial treatments are confined largely to universities and research clinics." (*ibid.* p.35). He sees as barriers: training, funding, poor accountability for outcomes, and a lack of an FDA-like approval system for such treatments.

The lack of strategic planning in how trained school mental health personnel are deployed to maximize an efficient prevention-intervention infrastructure remains a barrier to the model prescribed in this chapter. Furthermore, there is a lack of interdisciplinary research on this and other applied school mental health issues. For example, too frequently school owned mental health professionals are marginalized and not included in the research and analysis of prevention-intervention mental health service systems (Adelman & Taylor, 2000).

It has been shown that training can change practice and practice can change training (Canter & Gorin, 2001). Federal and state policies and local practice can change both. Laws and policies over the last quarter century have moved our children with serious emotional disorders from ineffective, restrictive institutions to the schoolhouse. These children are now moving from segregated special education schools and classrooms into regular classrooms with same-age peers. Special education law (P.L. 94-142, 1975) and its most recent revision (1997) gave children with disabilities civil rights to free and appropriate public education within the *least restrictive environment.*

The 1997 revision required more aggressive implementation of *least restrictive environment* and behavioral intervention plans to keep these children in school with their peers. These rights have again changed the face of schools, placing greater demands on regular educators; and successful inclusion programming requires a comprehensive, supportive infrastructure for both teachers and their students. However the lack of adequate funding and infrastructure, including insufficient numbers of school mental health providers within each state, remain barriers to success (Koyanigi & Gaines, 1993). Inclusion did change training. It required greater pre-service emphasis on addressing behavior within the regular education classroom and on consultation, using functional assessments of behavior, and greater use of training for school staff in positive behavioral supports. Recognizing this issue, training programs began to better address the consultation and training needs required to ensure the success of inclusive special education. Policy trends change pre-service training and effective practice has, slowly, begun to change schools. As part of this school-wide change it became apparent that regular classroom environmental factors could be modified to reduce behavior problems with non-disabled children, thus decreasing the number of children referred to be categorized as disabled. For example, practice has changed the state of Iowa's structure for serving children with academic and behavioral problems, reducing labeling children for

**Table 1.**

**Recommended Professional to Student Ratio and Estimated Number of Employed School Counselors, Psychologists & Social Workers**

| Recommended Professional: Student Ratio* | Estimated Number Employed | Estimated National Average** |
|---|---|---|
| One School Counselor for 250 students | 52,000 | 1: 1000 |
| One School Psychologist for 1000 students | 31,000 | 1: 1700 |
| One School Social Worker for 2,000 students | 14,000 | 1: 3700 |

**Minimum standard for one professional to total student population in service area.*
***Estimate based on total school age population of 52 million children and youth (2000-2001 school year).*

special education placements (Canter & Gorin, 2001).

Another barrier to service is the lack of these professionals employed by the nation's schools. Recommended ratios of professionals to student populations have been established for each of the three professions and are listed in Table 1. These minimum ratio standards are based on ideal school populations where 80 to 90% of the students are socially and academically able learners and 10-15% of students are "at-risk" of academic and psychosocial problems. In this hypothetical school 3-5% of the students may have functionally disabling behavioral or emotional problems.

These professional minimal standard ratios are rarely achieved in our nation's public schools. Furthermore, as minimal standards for ideal student populations, they are not designed to address the complex issues in schools that have high concentrations of students living in poverty and concentrations of children with identified special education needs. Under high concentrations of needs the recommended ratios are, for example one school psychologist for every 100 children with special needs and one social worker for 350 children in schools with high populations of children with special needs and poverty, language difference and other issues. Self-contained special schools, alternative schools and day treatment centers should consider a 1:50 ratio for both school psychologists and social workers. Therefore in a school where 80% of its students are receiving free or reduced lunch and 15% receiving special education services, the school social and psychological staffing ratio would need to be more than double the recommended minimal standard. Minimal standards are also inadequate to address the new crisis intervention needs related to both school violence and terrorism.

There are insufficient data sets for determining an accurate number of these three school mental health professions. The American School Counseling Association has 13,000 members, however many more counselors are employed in the schools. Some states prescribe a ratio of one counselor for every 500 students. The average is reported to be approximately 1:1000, which would result in an estimated 52,000 nationally if that ratio were evenly distributed among all K-12 grades (Institute of Medicine, 1997). The National Association of School Psychologists has 22,000 members and it is estimated that there are about 31,000 school psychologists serving school children across the United States (Thomas, 2001). Using this number, the ratio of school psychologists to students is presently about 1:1700. The U.S. Department of Education reports that there are 13,937 school social workers serving students within special education (USDOE, 2000). The ratio is calculated to be 1:3700.

Some states, such as Connecticut, have positive ratios of school mental health professionals to students and also established school health clinics (www. healthyschools.org, 2000). Connecticut has a school psychologist's ratio of 1:700 students and an additional 51 state supported school health clinics. There are only four states that approach the 1:1000 minimal recommended ratio of school psychologists to students (Curtis *et al.*, 1999).

Each of these three professions over the past three decades has moved progressively from a model of training for diagnosis and treatment to training for *systems change* with a strong emphasis on prevention, consultation and systemic reorientation. Cultural competence and alignment with family systems are also more strongly emphasized. This change has resulted in the production of a cadre of young professionals who are skilled to do far more than the routine role of refer-diagnose-treat, a system that labels children for special education services that focus only on deficit treatment. Even legislators are mandating a different professional service model in which these professionals, hired using federal dollars, provide preventive counseling and consultation services rather than merely diagnostic services and menial paperwork (Jackson-Lee, 2001).

Prevention is clearly a focus of pre-service training among these professions and is also a priority of their professional association's standards and resolutions (for example, see NASP, 2000). The emphasis on prevention, system reform and consultation are found in the *Blueprint for Training and Practice II* (Ysseldyke *et al.*, 1997) and other professional documents highlighting the importance of providing a cadre of mental health prevention/intervention specialists in the schools who have the ability to assist schools in changing how they educate and prepare children for life.

## Recommendations

School-based service programs that are planned using the public health framework (modified for schools) are beginning to show promise (Woodruff, *et al.*, 2000; Dwyer & Bernstein, 1998). It is becoming far more common across systems to utilize teams when addressing both universal prevention and intervention and the same should occur in our training institutions, both in courses and field placements for practicum and internship experiences. Clinical professionals, including child psychiatrists and psychologists should be provided opportunities to train collaboratively in school settings, participating on student service teams and developing role and responsibility plans with school mental health staff. Intensive interventions are - primarily - the purview of clinicians and these interventions may be best delivered in the school and the home by clinical mental health providers.

School pupil services mental health professionals are trained and credentialed to address child and adolescent behavior and emotional problems as those problems relate to academic learning and social adjustment. They are experts in functional behavioral assessments and analyses necessary for addressing the interaction effects of, for example, learning disabilities and adolescent depression. These school personnel can team with clinicians and provide behavioral observations to monitor treatment. School psychologists and others are skilled in examining the interplay between anxiety disorders, depression, conduct disorder, or the effects of medications on a child's socio-cognitive abilities within the classroom and ability to generalize a therapeutic cognitive strategy. School-based mental health professionals, such as school psychologists, are trained to provide consultation, brief therapies, psychological counseling, structured observations, functional and curriculum-based assessments, training in classroom accommodations for staff to address multiple types of disabilities, including attention-deficit hyperactivity disorder. They can identify barriers to learning within the child and within their environment and design and monitor behavioral plans. They are recognized for their ability to train teachers and other educational personnel in growth enhancing classroom management. In addition, they have been shown to be effective in problem-solving consultation, in training and supervising violence reduction programs of conflict resolution and peer mediation, and in improving school climate (Bear, Minke & Thomas, 1997). Using refer-question-consult models they identify and address early the needs of children on the trajectory of failure (Knoff, 1996). Utilizing early, targeted sets of coordinated intensive interventions, clinicians and school psychologists, counselors and social workers can partner to best serve the child and family. Their skills should be incorporated into school-community mental health teams.

These teams should identify service plans based on the child and family service needs. Access to effective services should be a primary focus for all professional teams. A child whose functional problems are severe and affect multiple areas of function should have available quality intensive interventions that can address all the child's needs. When such comprehensive services are not available, the child receives insufficient interventions and very frequently remains unsuccessful. Teaming enables monitoring and evaluation of interventions to best determine their positive effect size on the targeted behaviors and needs. The team can quickly respond to both a crisis and a failed or ineffectively applied intervention. They can evaluate efficacy and fidelity of interventions applied in the natural environment of the school. The team approach is highlighted in the federal document *Safeguarding Our Children: An Action Guide* (Dwyer & Osher, 2000).

The public health model applied to the schools has shown merit. Yet none of these effective model programs have been brought to scale. One reason is funding, however, the costs to society far-out weigh the cost of interventions. Another reason is the lack of cooperation among service systems and professionals in education and clinical mental health settings. Blending funding and directing more funding toward prevention is a policymaking task. Establishing positive partnerships among professions and better determining roles in the implementation of the public health model for mental health in school communities is the critical responsibility of the professions, their training programs, professional associations and the professionals in each community. Otherwise, the professions are part of the problem.

Professional associations need to aggressively support interprofessional collaboration both in pre-service preparation, internship placements and community practice. Professional associations must work together to examine existing practice, and to support continued professional development in proven practices for licensed/certified professionals.

Policymakers need to consider supporting the pre-service training of all children's mental health professions with a critical focus on incentives to recruit and retain racially and ethnically underrepresented groups. Research needs to examine all existing service systems for their mental health role and effectiveness. Presently, there is no accurate data collection with regard to how many children are receiving effective services from the over 90,000 counselors, school psychologists and social workers employed by schools.

Promotion of mental health and the prevention of mental health problems must be taught and its practice funded. The death rate among adolescents mandates that funding be shifted from emergency room treatment for gunshots to prevention of impulsive aggressive behavior. We must train for crisis prevention as well as crisis intervention.

Research is needed to compare effective systemic preventive interventions for application with cultural, economic and geographic groups. University training programs should utilize cooperative agreements to secure research funding and other incentives to replicate programs in natural settings and study the management models that enable bringing effective programs to scale. Universities should partner, more frequently, with families and community organizations (*e.g.* Mental Health Associations) to effect community change. More research is needed to look at the clinic vs. school based mental health service models. University preparation programs need to use technology more effectively in the training for the common factors among comprehensive prevention-intervention models. Such training needs to include elements of applicability including cost, staffing and training requirements as they relate to positive effect size.

Pre-service training in teaming skills should be required for all mental health professionals. Knowledge and skills among members must enable the team to provide the kind of direction and support needed for systemic and individualized academic and behavioral interventions. If there is no one on the team, whose competencies include the ability to translate behavioral and academic and systems research into practice, teams will be ineffective. If no one on the team knows how to effectively analyze school-community climate, environmental factors may remain toxic. Teams must have skills to redirect behavior, improve coping strategies, utilize positive behavioral supports in the classroom, manage group behavior, apply appropriate developmental and behavioral theory to individual problems and to school factors. Understanding and knowing how to respond to developmental psychopathology within the school setting is critical to a student support team's effectiveness.

Families, children and youth, our consumers, desire observable results. Intervention outcomes must be measured. What measures will treatment teams use when determining if interventions have *functional* outcomes? Improved social and academic functioning, measures of attendance, grades, discipline referrals, class-engaged time, and participation in extra-curricular activities, among others that schools already measure and parents value.

All professionals should be accountable to demonstrate required sets of skills according to their role and their profession's competency standards. Systems should make in-service training available to bring existing professionals up to those standards. Competency standards should be publicly known so that families and employers can better identify effective providers and effective service teams.

The Surgeon General identified the needs with regard to children's mental health and identified effective solutions. It is our responsibility to fix what we know is broken, to prevent ineffective services from continuing, and to replace the ineffective with effective programs in every school community.

## References


Adelman, H. S. (2001). The Policy Leadership Cadre for Mental Health in Schools: Resource and Reference Position. Los Angeles CA: Center for Mental Health in the Schools. Department of Psychology, UCLA.

Adelman, H. S. (1996) Restructuring educational support services and integrating community resources: beyond the full service school model. *School Psychology Review.* 25: 431-445.

Adelman H. and Taylor, L. (2000). A sampling of outcome findings from interventions relevant to addressing barriers to learning. Los Angeles, CA: Mental Health in the Schools Training and Technical Assistance Center. Department of Psychology, UCLA.

Adelman H. and Taylor, L. (1999). Mental health in schools and system restructuring. *Clinical Psychology Review.* 19: 137-163.

Albee, G.W. and Gullotta, T.P. (1997). Primary Prevention Works. Thousand Oaks CA: SAGE Publications.

Allensworth, D. and Kolbe, L. (1987). The comprehensive school health program: Exploring an expanded concept. *Journal of School Health*, 57: 409-412.

American School Counselor Association. (1997). National Standards for School Counseling Programs of the American School Counselor Association. Alexandria VA

Bear, G.G., Minke, K.M., and Thomas, A. (Eds.) (1997). Children's needs II: Development, problems and alternatives. Bethesda MD: National Association of School Psychologists.

Burns, B.J., Costello, E.J., Angold, A., *et al.* (1995) Children's mental health services use across service sectors. *Health Affairs*, 14, 147-159

Canter, A. and Gorin, S. (2001). Mile high at the summit: NASP launches strategic plan. *Communiqué*, 30: pp. 1, 6-7. National Association of School Psychologists.

Center for Mental Health Services (July, 1999). Matrix of Evidence-based Prevention Interventions. Rockville MD: Substance Abuse and Mental Health Services Administration, U.S. DHHS.

Children's Defense Fund, (1996). The State of America's Children: Yearbook, 1996. Washington DC.

Curtis, M.J., Hunley, S.A., Walker, K.J., and Baker, A.C. (1999) Demographic characteristics and professional practices in school psychology. *School Psychology Review*, 28: pp.104-116.

Curtis M.J. and Stollar, S.A. (1995). System-level consultation and organizational change. In A. Thomas and J. Grimes, Eds. Best Practices in School Psychology. Washington DC: National Association of School Psychologists.

Dryfoos, J. (1994). Full-service schools: A revolution in health and social services for children, youth, and families. San Francisco, CA: Josey-Bass, Inc.

Dwyer, K.P. & Bernstein, R. (1998). Mental health in the schools: Linking islands of hope in a sea of despair. *School Psychology Review*, 27: pp. 277-286.

Dwyer, K.P. and Osher, D. (2000). Safeguarding Our Children: An Action Guide. Washington D.C. U.S. Departments of Education & Justice, American Institutes for Research.

Elias, M.J., & Tobias, S.E. (1996) Social Problem Solving: Interventions in the Schools. New York, NY: Guilford Press.

Elliott, D.S. (ed). (1998). Blueprint for violence prevention. Book 10: Promoting Alternative Thinking Strategies (PATHS). Boulder, CO: Institute of Behavioral Science.

Fagan, T. Sachs Wise, P. (2000). School Psychology: Past, Present and Future. (Second Edition). Bethseda MD: National Association of School Psychologists.

Fagan, T. (1995). Trends in the history of school psychology in the United States. In A. Thomas, and J. Grimes (Eds.) Best Practices in School Psychology III. (pp. 59-67). Washington DC: National Association of School Psychologists.

Felson, R. (1996). Mass media effects on violent behavior. *Annual Review of Sociology*, 22: 103-128.

Forness, S. (2001). Schools and identification of mental health needs. Report of the Surgeon General's Conference on Children's Mental Health: A national agenda. Washington DC: Department of Health and Human Services.

Greenberg, M.T., Domitrovich, C., and Bumbarger, B. (2001). The prevention of mental disorders in school-aged children: Current state of the field. *Prevention and Treatment*, 4: Article 1.

Hamburg, M.A. (1998). Youth violence is a public health concern. In D.S. Elliott, B.A. Hamburg and K.R.Williams (Eds.). Violence in American Schools: A New Perspective. New York: Cambridge University Press. (pp. 31-54)

Hess, R. and Copeland, E.P. (1997). Stress. In, G.G. Bear, K.M. Minke, and A.Thomas (Eds.) Children's needs II: Development, problems and needs. Bethesda MD: National Association of School Psychologists. pp. 293-304.

Hollis, J., & Wantz, R.A. (1997). Counselor preparation 1993-1995: Vol. II Status, Trends and Implications. 8th Edition. Muncie IN: Accelerated Development Press.

Institute of Medicine. (1997). Schools & Health: Our Nation's Investment. Committee on Comprehensive School Health in Grades K-12. Washington DC: National Academy Press.

Jackson-Lee, S. (2001). HR. 75 Give a kid a chance: Omnibus mental health bill of 2001. 107th U.S. Congress.

Kazdin, A.E. (1991). Prevention of conduct disorder. The Prevention of Mental Disorders: Progress, Problems & Prospects. Washington DC: National Institute of Mental Health.

Kelleher, K.J., McInerny, T.K., Gardner, W.P., *et al.* (1999) Increasing identification of psychosocial problems: 1979-1997. University of Pennsylvania Medical School Consensus Conference on Attention Deficit Hyperactivity Disorder. Philadelphia PA: kelleherkj@msx.upmc.edu

Knitzer, J., Steinberg, Z., and Fleisch, B. (1990). At the Schoolhouse Door: An Examination of Programs and Policies for Children with Behavior and Emotional Problems. New York: Bank Street College of Education.

Knoff, H.M. (1996). The interface of school, community and health care reform: Organizational directions toward effective services for children. *School Psychology Review*, 25: 446-464.

Knoff, H.M., and Batsche, G.M. (1995). Project ACHIEVE: Analyzing a school reform process for at-risk and underachieving students. *School Psychology Review*, 24, 579-603.

Koyanagi, C. and Gaines, S. (1993). All systems failure: An examination of the results of neglecting the needs of children with serious emotional disorder. Alexandria, VA: National Mental Health Association.

Kumpfer, K.L., DeMarsh, J. and Child, W.P. (1988). Strengthening Families Training Manuals. Salt Lake City: University of Utah, Social Research Institute.

Learning First Alliance (2001). Every Child Learning: Safe and Supportive schools. Washington DC.

Lodge, .D. (1998) California's Healthy Start: Strong Families, Strong Communities for Student Success. Santa Barbara CA: California Department of Education.

Making the Grade (1995) Issues in Financing School-based Health Centers: A Guide for State Officials. Washington, DC: The George Washington University.

Manderscheid, R.W. and Henderson, M.J. Mental Health United States, 1998. Rockville, MD: U.S. Department of Health & Human Services.

Mandalwitz, M. (2001). School Social Work Association of America.

Marx, E. and Wooley, S. (Eds.) (1998). Health is Academic. New York: Teachers College Press.

Nastasi, B.K., Varjas, K., and Bernstein, R. (1998). Exemplary Mental Health Programs: School Psychologists as Mental Health Service Providers. Washington, DC: National Association of School Psychologists.

National Alliance of Pupil Services Organizations (1994). Pupil Services: A Position Statement. Washington, DC.

National Association of School Based Health Clinics (Personal communication September, 2000).

National Association of School Psychologists. (2000). Professional Conduct Manual: Principles of Ethics; Guidelines for the Provision of School Psychological Services. Bethesda, MD.

National Association of School Psychologists. (2000). Standards for School Psychology: Training Programs; Field Placement; Credentialing Standards. Bethesda, MD.

National Association of Social Workers. (1992). Specialty Certification for the Experienced MSW School Social Worker. Washington DC.

National Research Council & Institute of Medicine (2001). Getting to Positive Outcomes for Children in Childcare. Washington DC: National Academy Press.

National Research Council & Institute of Medicine (2000). From Neurons to Neighborhoods: The Science of Early Childhood Development. Washington DC: National Academy Press.

National Research Council & Institute of Medicine. (1999). Risk and Opportunities: Synthesis of Studies on Adolescence. Washington DC: National Academy Press.

Prothrow-Stith, D. Share what you know! Keynote Address, National Association of School Psychologists 33rd Annual Convention. Washington DC. Author.

Reschly, D.J. and Ysseldyke, J.E. (1995). School psychology paradigm shift. (p17-31). In Thomas, A., and Grimes, J. (Eds.) Best Practices in School Psychology III. Washington DC: National Association of School Psychologists.

SBHCNet. (2000). State Resources: State & City reports: Connecticut School-based Health Centers. Washington DC: Making the Grade, George Washington University.

Shaffer, D. *et al.* (1996). Psychiatric diagnosis in child and adolescent suicide. *Archives of General Psychiatry*, 53: 339-348.

Shure, M.B. (1997). Interpersonal cognitive problem solving: Primary prevention of early high-risk behaviors in the preschool and primary years. In Albee, G.W. and Gullotta, T.P. (Eds.), Primary Prevention Works (pp. 167-188). Thousand Oaks, CA: Sage.

Thomas, A. (2001). School psychology numbers. Report to the Delegate Assembly, July 2001. Washington DC: National Association of School Psychologists.

U.S. Departments of Education (2000). Twenty-second Annual Report to Congress on the Implementation of the Individuals with Disabilities Education Act. Washington DC.

U.S. Department of Health and Human Services (2001). Youth Violence: A Report of the Surgeon General. Washington DC: Government Printing Office.

U.S. Department of Health and Human Services (1999). Mental Health: A Report of the Surgeon General. Washington DC: Government Printing Office.

U.S. Department of Health and Human Services (1996). Trends in the Well-being of America's Children and Youth: 1996.

Walker, H.M. (1999). Three-tiered model of school-wide discipline strategies. In J. Sprague & H.M. Walker (Eds.) Community-based Prevention and Intervention Training Manual. Institute on Violence and Destructive Behavior, University of Oregon.

Walker, H.M. and Rankin, R. (1983). Assessing the behavioral expectations and demands of less restrictive settings. *School Psychology Review*, 12: 274-284.

Weisz, J.R. (2001). State of the evidence on treatments for children and the research to practice gap. Report of the Surgeon General's Conference on Children's Mental Health: A National Agenda. Washington DC: Department of Health and Human Services.

Woodruff, D.W., *et al.* (1999). The role of education in a system of care: Effectively children with emotional and behavioral disorders. Systems of Care: Promising Practices in Children's Mental Health, 1998 Series, Volume III. Washington D.C.: Center for Effective Collaboration and Practice, American Institutes for Research.

Wright, D. (1996). Functional Behavioral Assessment and Interventions. Sacramento CA: California Department of Education.

Ysseldyke, J., *et al.* (1997). School Psychology: A Blueprint for Training and Practice II. Bethesda MD: National Association of School Psychologists.

Ysseldyke, J., *et al.* (1984). School Psychology: A Blueprint for Training and Practice. Minneapolis MN: National School Psychology Inservice Training Network, University of Minnesota.

## Developmental and Prevention Issues – Children

**Barry S. Zuckerman, M.D.,**
**Boston University Medical Center**

I have spent most of my career as a somewhat atypical pediatrician. I have gone beyond the usual disciplinary boundaries that include a broad mental health perspective. This reflects my primary concern for going beyond just treating the presenting symptoms but also meeting the comprehensive needs of the child and family. That is, to have a goal of attaining and maintaining a trajectory of health growth and development for all patients.

It became clear that health and mental health are intertwined and are integral to the process of determining physical and mental well-being, social competence and providing the basis for affective learning in addition to pediatric medicine. As a result, I draw heavily on the knowledge bases of child development, social cognition, life course studies and the field of mental health.

In the mental health arena recently there has been heavy emphasis on the importance of prevention. When we think about the spectrum of preventive interventions whether it is in the context of sensitive periods of development and vicissitudes of normal transitions periods or situations in which the vicissitudes are excessive and could cause great harm, prevention interventions are possible and can be very effective. Prevention becomes a large framework for organizing and integrating a broad therapeutic approach to a humane and meaningful care of children and their families.

A National Academy of Sciences report laid out what we know about impact of early experiences on brain development. Those early experiences have an impact on later behavior, and also on the developing brain. One point that they mentioned is that parental mental health has a huge impact on children. Depression is prevalent; and domestic violence equally prevalent if not more so and maybe more malignant. Thus the notion of a two-generational approach to child health and well-being is critical to the efficacy of certain child interventions.

There is an overlap between mental health and normal physical development. The report looked at adult health disparities, and traced them back to child health and development and cognitive disparities, and basically integrated knowledge about environment and early childhood. Some of these adult disparities probably had their beginnings in the first few years of life because of those impacts and the social context on a child's brain and behavior.

It makes all the sense in the world and is consistent with my experience as a pediatrician, watching how children progress over the years, to ask what are the relative contributions of stressors and protective factors in shaping the child's trajectory of growth and development.

We have learned that although mind and body interact, there can be disconnects between the observable behavior of the child and the physiological functioning of the body for example, among those children who are quiet and shy in a novel situation, blood pressure and heart rate go up even though the behavior appears unperturbed. These children seem to be vulnerable to depression unless their vulnerability is recognized and handled appropriately. On the other hand there are other children in novel situations who appear very excitable and highly active whose blood pressure and heart rate are unperturbed. Current studies examine whether or not these differences signify vulnerability to future mental disorders such as depression, anxiety or physical disorders such as hypertension, or diabetes.

The integration of physiology, behavior, and mental health: it's all there and sooner or later we have to come to grips with it. We do more in a research setting than in its application to practice; but as that knowledge progresses, there's no sense in doing the research because we won't be able to apply it in our present models.

Two other streams, preventive mental health and the movement from the education community about entering school ready to learn, offer opportunities for research and practice. Two programs address the inferences and have to do with systems change, not problem solving in a linear way. If all factors are interrelated, though, we need multiple strategic interventions to make a difference. Also, it turns out, small things can have a big impact.

The best example is a program called Reach Out and Read where pediatricians promote literacy in the office. Books offer a way to discuss issues, and reading makes bedtime easier. The primary care provider gives simple recommendations about reading aloud to children at every visit and provides a new book at each visit up to five years. That is about nine or 10 books by the time the child starts kindergarten. They start as small books: board books babies can chew on, brightly colored books about familiar objects— babies, family members and animals.

How does that change what we do? It changes people's mindset to get people thinking about what we can do. We always thought the most important thing parents can do is read, but that never got translated. With these books parents are four to eight times more likely to read to kids. That has translated to improved language scores in low income children. Home interventions, give a book, and the parent can do the work. One thousand sites nationally gave away a couple of million books. I think it started to change pediatrics and get pediatricians to think about developmental issues. That is much different from a developmental assessment, if you start asking parents when can they read, when do they recognize letters.

We started a witness to violence program, as an example of prevention. We do counseling for children who witness domestic violence. I got tired of reading about mothers being killed and children huddled in corner but physically unmarred. As part of prevention, we started training police, with ten one- and a half-hour sessions. It has been a marvelous experience. They care about kids, and we give skills on how to speak to kids. We see them as outreach workers who now have language to talk to kids and know how to refer. The police say it helps change their behavior.

How do we have an impact based on our knowledge? How do we use our skill to communicate with others? The police are not who we usually think about, but I think we need changes in all our systems because families have changed. Community police have changed their paradigm to meet needs of people in their community.

With parental illness, when we think about our efforts as pediatricians, or any of home visiting intensive efforts around children at risk, one group of mothers who don't react well are those with post-traumatic stress disorder, who cannot make relationships and cannot benefit from outreach services. I don't know what will help, but these mothers are numb to their feeling: they are damaged. Whether it is childhood or sexual abuse in the past, current physical or sexual abuse — they need help. We reach a lot of depressed mothers, but can't reach mothers with post-traumatic stress syndrome.

There is little data about the impact of post-traumatic stress on parenting, or the impact of interventions on parenting. Now we have six post-traumatic stress child centers and I think this is a way of moving the field.

We now have three legal aid lawyers in primary care settings and specialty clinics to make sure families have basic safety, health, food, and housing needs met. Without basic needs met, parenting is difficult, but if the goal is the well being of children why not do this? We could send them away to legal aid clinics. They were not doing it, so we went ahead on our own.

By bringing in early childhood intervention, by bringing in lawyers, that's the way we change a system. We don't change by all of us thinking the same, but by bringing in different people who give us new ideas and new ways of doing things. We have spent a lot of time trying to figure out how to evaluate the legal aid program. If they are getting food, that's better. This really is an issue of social justice, not outcomes research.

The largest experiment in prevention is a program called Healthy Steps funded by the Commonwealth Fund. It now includes about 27 practices: academic, HMOs, private offices and clinics, a randomized trial of enhanced prevention approaches in a pediatric setting. This is a new system of pediatric care, with an early childhood specialist in practice, not for practice but for prevention. This is a new person who will see parents for 30-40 minutes each visit, do home visits, and be available by phone. Johns Hopkins is making an independent evaluation.

Some of the non-specific aspects of the psychotherapeutic context are important for all of the interventions that pediatricians might do. Hopefully stories about some of this work have inferences for how to think about prevention, the role of child psychiatry training, and practice in the future.

## Advances in the Care of the Elderly

**Dan G. Blazer, M.D., Ph.D.**
**JP Gibbons Professor of Psychiatry and Behavioral Sciences**
**Duke University Medical Center**

### Introduction: The Aging Imperative

Geriatric psychiatry came of age during the past two decades.[1,2] The American Board of Psychiatry and Neurology, as of 1991, now offers a certificate of added qualifications in geriatric psychiatry (well over 2000 certificates offered thus far). Multiple subspecialty journals have emerged, such as the *American Journal of Geriatric Psychiatry*, the *International Journal of Psychogeriatrics* and the *International Journal of Geriatric Psychiatry. The American Association of Geriatric Psychiatry* includes over 1500 persons on its roles and over 1000 persons attend the annual meeting. One reason for the dramatic increase in interest in the elderly is the current aging imperative. Our society is aging and the impact upon our society in terms of income distribution and health care resources, among other factors, has been dramatic.

Of the 275+ million persons counted during the Unites States census of 2000, nearly 35 million, or 13% of the population, is 65+ years of age.[3] The mean age in the United States is now 36 years. Even more astounding, over four million, or 1.6% of the US population and 12.5% of the 65+ age group, are 85+ years of age. These oldest old among us are projected to reach 20 million by the year 2050 and to make up 5% of the US population at that time. The "old-old" are more likely to experience poverty, to have less education, and to receive far more federal transfer payments. Over 50% of nursing home residents in the US are 80 years old or older, representing a cost of over 30 billion dollars per year.[4] At least one-half of these residents are placed in nursing homes because of neuropsychiatric disorders such as Alzheimer's disease and the resulting behavioral complications such as behavioral disturbances.

The size of the elderly population in the US is expected to double during the next 30 years, reaching 70 million by the year 2030.[3] Most of these elders are women (58%) and white (84%). Women should continue to survive longer than men, yet the racial/ethnic composition of the elderly will change dramatically over the next few decades. Currently, 8% of elders are non-Hispanic black, 2% are non-Hispanic Asian and Pacific Islander, and less than 1% are non-Hispanic American Indian/Alaska natives. Hispanic elders make up

6% the 65+ age group. By 2050, the percentage of white, non-Hispanic elders will decline to 64% and Hispanic persons will account for 16% (a growth of 11 million persons) with non-Hispanic blacks accounting for 12%.

In 1900 the life expectancy at birth was 49 years.[3] In 1997 the life expectancy at birth was 79 years for women and 74 years for men. Persons who survive to age 65 can expect to live an average of nearly 18 more years. Life expectancy of persons who survive to age 85 is 7 years for women and 6 years for men. If an older person develops a psychiatric disorder, that disorder not only may become chronic, but the years of life which are associated with a decreased quality of life because of psychiatric morbidity are substantial. In addition, with increasing age, the great majority of older persons with psychiatric disorders also experience comorbid physical illnesses.

Health care expenditures for older persons are staggering given their annual income, and only the availability of universal health insurance for elders through Medicare and Medicaid (which supports much long-term care) insures a modicum of reasonable care to older adults for physical and psychiatric disorders. Of the 1.3 trillion dollars spent on health care in the US annually, Medicare (which predominantly provides resources to the elderly) accounts for 20% and Medicaid (a significant proportion going to long-term care) accounts for 14%).[3] Medicare is projected to account for nearly 4% of the gross domestic product by the year 2025. The average annual expenditure on health care in 1996 was $5,864 among persons 65-69, $9,414 among persons 75-79 and $16,465 among persons 85+. Older persons living in institutions incurred $38,906 in annual health care expense (64% being for nursing home care). The top 5% of enrollees with the highest expenditures incurred 37% of all health care expenses among the elderly. Twenty-nine percent of all health care expenditures went to inpatient care with 10% to going to skilled nursing home care and home care. In 1998, households headed by older persons in the bottom fifth of the income distribution spent an average of $1,654 per year on health care out of pocket (13% of their annual income) compared to $3,614 among households in the top fifth of the income distribution (9% of their annual income).

In summary, the elderly are the predominant recipients of health care in the United States and much of this care, especially long-term care, results from the direct and indirect costs of psychiatric disorders. For these reasons, much attention has been directed in recent years to the two disorders in late life which account for most of the burden in psychiatric impairment, late life depression and Alzheimer's disease.[5, 6]

## The Mental Health Imperative

The mental health imperative for seniors in the United States might be summarized with three "Ps" and illustrated by late life depression and Alzheimer's disease. Psychiatric disorders are *profound* in their impact upon the economic well-being and quality of life among seniors. As noted above, psychiatric disorders account for at least one-half of the morbidity in long term care and are the prime reason for admission among the same proportion. Psychiatric disorders among seniors are *preventable* by avoiding or delaying onset, reducing the initial burden of symptoms and reducing functional impairment over time. For example, recent studies have demonstrated that early intervention to treat major depression in the elderly significantly reduces the risk of recurrence and dysfunction over time.[7] Evidence has emerged that the progression of Alzheimer's disease can be significantly retarded by the use of anticholinesterase inhibitors.[8] Finally, elders with psychiatric disorders are often *precluded* from adequate mental health care due to inadequate funding of research, training and service provision. Care for psychiatric disorders in late life has experienced a similar discrimination in funding through Medicare as has the care of these disorders been grossly under funded by health maintenance organizations. Specifically, Medicare offers no general outpatient prescription drug coverage and limits inpatient hospital days.[9]

## Late Life Depression

The novelist William Styron experienced a severe and prolonged episode of depression as he entered late life. He describes the pain as a darkness visible. "Depression is a disorder of mood, so mysteriously painful and elusive in the way it becomes known to the self - to the mediating intellect - as to verge close to being beyond description. It thus remains nearly incomprehensible to those who have not experienced it in its extreme mood, although the gloom, "the blues" which people go through occasionally and associate with the general hassle of everyday existence are of such prevalence that they do give many individuals a hint of the illness in its catastrophic form."[10]

Depressive symptoms increase with increasing age, though the diagnosis of major depression may actually decrease.[11, 12] Many symptoms of depression are especially frequent and persistent among older persons, such as sadness (over 20% of community dwelling elders complain of persistent sadness over one week and nearly 15% complain of persistent loneliness).[13] The discrepancy between the burden of symptoms and the diagnosis of the disorder in community samples should not limit the interest in the burden of depression in the elderly. To provide one example of the challenge, suicide rates are higher in late life than at any other age, and are especially high among elderly white males.[14] In one study, the investigators found a four-fold increase in the odds of dying over a follow-up of 15 months if persons 55+ years of age experienced a mood disorder in a community sample.[15] This association of depression and mortality in late life has been confirmed in Australia[16] and Japan.[17]

Many potential control variables are associated with both depression and mortality, the primary ones being age, medical illness, cognitive impairment and functional impairment. Depression has been shown in numerous studies to be associated with medical illness.[18, 19] Depression is also known to be associated with cognitive impairment, especially via co-morbidity with Alzheimer's Disease and vascular dementia.[20] The relationship between depression and functional impairment has also been well established in the literature, with the association suggesting a complementary feedback mechanism, *i.e.*, in longitudinal studies depression can precede functional impairment or functional impairment can precede depression.[21] Functional impairment, in turn, is a known risk for increased mortality.[22] Depression is also known to be associated with smoking, impaired social support, unmarried status and poor self-rated health.[23 - 26] These factors, in turn, have been associated with increased mortality.[26, 27]

Elders experiencing depression are much higher users of health care services.[28] In a four-year prospective cohort study of 2558 elderly subjects in a large staff-model health maintenance organization in Seattle, Washington, depressive symptoms were common and associated with increases in the cost of general health services. The depressed were more likely to use outpatient services, to be admitted to the hospital, twice as likely to visit an ER and used a higher number of prescription medications in controlled analyses. Depressed elders accumulated more health care costs whether they had no other chronic conditions or whether they had many chronic conditions.

Though effective treatment of depression is undoubtedly far from universal among older persons, one barometer of the burden of depression is the marked increase in use of antidepressant medications in recent years. From 1986 to 1996 the use of antidepressants by an aging cohort of elders in North Carolina nearly quadrupled (from less than 4% to 12%).[29] This trend mirrored a general trend in our society with the introduction of the selective serotonin reuptake inhibitors and related compounds. What renders the finding remarkable, however, is that the increase occurred within an aging cohort (aging from 65+ to 75+ years over the ten years of follow-up). The increase was not uniform across races (with a four-fold higher use by whites compared to African Americans, even controlling for depressive symptoms and socioeconomic status).

Given the public health burden of late life depression, a consensus conference on late life depression was convened nearly ten years ago to review the extant literature and make recommendations.[5] Since that time, many basic and clinical research projects have been fielded to explore the pathophysiology of late life depression and to test intervention strategies which have proven effective earlier in life. Investigators, for example, have explored depression associated with subcortical white matter hyperintensities found with magnetic resonance imaging. They have labeled this depressive variant in late life as "vascular depression".[30] Vascular depression is more frequent in oldest old, with late age of onset, nonpsychotic depression. Family history of depression is somewhat less frequent. Anhedonia and functional disability, in contrast, are more frequent.

Other investigators have expanded this construct, suggesting that the portion of the brain specifically affected by these vascular lesions relevant to late life depression is executive function.[31] Executive dysfunction, including disturbances in planning, sequencing, organizing, and abstracting, has been associated with late life depression. Executive dysfunction, in contrast to memory impairment, is associated with late onset depression in late life and also with relapse and recurrence. Executive dysfunction may result from disruption of the cortico-striatal-pallido-thalamo-cortical pathway (the function of which is modulated by the raphe nuclei, locus ceruleus and ventral tegmentum).

Treatment regimes which have proved effective in preventing recurrence of major depression in younger adults have been applied to older adults in the ambulatory setting.[7] By combining interpersonal psychotherapy with ongoing use of antidepressant medications, the frequency of recurrence of major depression was reduced significantly. These studies mark a significant change in the attitude toward aggressive therapy of late life depression. When Salzman reviewed the controlled clinical trials of antidepressant medications among the elderly for the 1991 consensus conference, the studies were quite limited.[32] Since that time, however, over 100 published reports of controlled trials, many of which include the oldest old, have appeared.[33] The therapeutic nihilism which persisted in psychiatry for many years regarding the treatment of late life depression has largely disappeared among academic psychiatrists.

## Alzheimer's Disease

Disabling memory loss may begin in mid-life, but it is much more frequent in persons older than age 75 years than it is in persons between ages 65 and 74. Prevalence estimates from community samples of memory impairment are generally 5%–15%, with most investigators estimating memory impairment in at least 10% of persons older than age 65 years in the community and in 30%–50% of institutional residents.[34] Alzheimer's disease, the most common disorder contributing to the dementia syndrome, has been estimated to be prevalent in 6-8% of community-based persons older than age 65 years, with more than 30% of persons age 85 years or older experiencing Alzheimer's disease. Prevalence estimates of Alzheimer's disease include both mild and severe cases, so significant memory impairment may be found in only a proportion of persons identified as having Alzheimer's disease in community samples. Other causes of memory loss include vascular dementia, Lewy body dementia, dementia associated with Parkinson's disease and alcohol related dementias. Yet the majority of dementias among the elderly are caused by Alzheimer's disease, either in whole or in part.

Memory loss is usually progressive with the prevalence doubling every 5 years after the age of 60 years.[34] Until age 75, the life expectancy of persons experiencing Alzheimer's disease or vascular dementia is reduced by about one-half. After age 75, life expectancy is less affected by memory loss. Even those persons who have Alzheimer's disease or vascular dementias may experience significant decline over an interval, only to enter a "plateau" in functioning for a subsequent interval that may last for many months.

More than 50% of persons experiencing chronic memory loss will, at autopsy, exhibit the changes of Alzheimer's disease only. The next most common contributors to the syndrome are the vascular dementias. Clinically and pathophysiologically, it is difficult to disaggregate the vascular dementias. (For example, it is difficult to distinguish vascular dementia from Binswanger's disease.) Vascular dementia also frequently is comorbid with Alzheimer's disease.[35] In contrast to Alzheimer's disease, however, vascular dementia is more common in males than in females. Many patients with Parkinson's disease develop brain changes late in the course of their disease similar to those changes found in Alzheimer's disease. Clinically, except for their parkinsonian symptoms, these patients cannot be distinguished from patients experiencing Alzheimer's disease. In addition, many patients with Alzheimer's disease exhibit changes in the substantia nigra at autopsy.

The primary risk factors for Alzheimer's disease are age and family history, with the prevalence of Alzheimer's, as mentioned previously, being an exponential function of age. Other risk factors for Alzheimer's disease include Down's syndrome, head trauma, and possibly lack of education. Genetic risk factors have received much attention in recent years, especially the relationship between the disease and apolipoprotein E (APOE) genotype.[36] The APOE genotype expresses itself in three alleles (2, 3, and 4). Persons with an APOE genotype of 4/4 are at much greater risk for developing Alzheimer's disease than are persons with a 2/2 genotype, with a range of risk between the most vulnerable (4/4) and the most protective (2/2). Much less frequent forms of Alzheimer's disease have been link to chromosome 12 among others. Most cases of Alzheimer's disease, however, cannot be attributed to one etiological agent. Male sex, hypertension, and possibly black race are risk factors for vascular dementia.

Recent advances in understanding the pathophysiology of Alzheimer's have been dramatic. Many pieces of the puzzle which lay scattered before have recently come together, suggesting not only more specific treatment strategies but also preventive strategies.[37] The relationship of cholesterol to Alzheimer's disease initially was noted through the identification of a susceptibility gene for Alzheimer's, namely the E4 variant of the apolipoprotein E gene noted above.[38] This gene encodes for a protein which carries cholesterol. More recently, investigators have found that the cholesterol-lowering statins may be especially protective against the development of Alzheimer's.[39] These scattered epidemiologic findings to date, however, have only lead to speculation regarding the pathophysiology of the disease.

Investigators have long suspected that the beta amyloid protein causes the brain degeneration in Alzheimer's. It now appears that cholesterol augments amyloid deposition. In another study, the cholesterol lowering drug simvastatin was demonstrated to lower amyloid peptides in vitro.[37, 40] Cells produce the peptide amyloid by clipping it out of a larger protein called APP (for amyloid precursor protein), with the aid of two enzymes, known as alpha and beta secretases. But APP is also cut by another enzyme, called gamma secretase. Because this enzyme breaks APP within the amyloid segment, it prevents production of the neurotoxic peptide. It appears that cholesterol lowering treatments inhibit amyloid beta protein formation by shifting the balance of the activities of these enzymes to favor gamma secretase.

These experiments pave an increasingly clear pathway to more specific therapy for Alzheimer's disease. For the present, however, clinicians are using a more distal and symptomatic therapy, anti-cholinesterase inhibition. Three such medications are currently available (or will be available) — donepezil (Aricept), rivastigmine (Exelon), and galantamine (Reminyl). The efficacy of these drugs appears to be dose related and their side effects are mild to moderate, with gastrointestinal symptoms being the most common. They are thought to improve or at least stabilize cognitive decline in Alzheimer's disease over the first year of therapy and to stabilize or slow the decline over succeeding years. Keeping patients at higher doses of the drugs appears to increase the effectiveness of the drugs. One encouraging finding is that the medications may have some of their most beneficial effects during the middle stages of the disease.[8]

Perhaps the most difficult aspect of the dementing disorders to treat is the behavioral disturbances, especially agitation and suspiciousness. The neuroleptics are the most effective psychotropics for controlling severe agitation, aggressive behavior, and psychoses. Most neuroleptics are effective but produce side effects, and, therefore, the selection of a drug is usually determined by the side-effect profile least adverse for a given patient. For this reason the new generation antipsychotic agents, such as olanzapine, quetiepine and risperidone are the preferred drugs at present.[41] The most troublesome side effects that ensue from using neuroleptic agents are postural hypotension (and the risk of falling) and tardive dyskinesia. Both of these adverse consequences of therapy appear to be less common when using the new generation antipsychotics.

## Looking to the Future

Despite the dramatic growth of the investigative base for the practice of geriatric psychiatry and the increasing availability of evidenced-based interventions for the most disabling disorders in late life, some believe that we are facing an upcoming crisis in the field.[42] Reporting results from a consensus conference, leaders in geriatric psychiatry project that the number of people in the United States over the age of 65 experiencing psychiatric disorders will increase from 4 million in 1970 to over 15 million in 2030. They further suggest that the current health care system serves mentally ill older adults poorly and is unprepared to meet this crisis. They note correctly that most elders experiencing psychiatric disorders do not seek nor are they referred to psychiatrists, much less geriatric psychiatrists. The quality of care they receive for their psychiatric disorders has been questioned.

In one study, the investigators found that 55% of internists believed themselves competent to diagnose depression in the elderly yet only 35% felt competent to prescribe medications.[43] Three-fourths of these physicians thought that depression was to be expected in older adults. In another study, fewer than 25% of patients with moderate to severe dementia were identified by general practitioners as having dementia.[44]

Perhaps one of the most critical areas of neglect in geriatric psychiatry is the neglect of the oldest old.[2] In the United States, the term "oldest old" was coined in 1984 to highlight the 85 plus age group as the largest growing age group in our society (as noted above).[4] Not only are these elders becoming more frequent in our society, they are becoming of more importance to psychiatry. Yet they remain difficult to study and are poorly understood by psychiatrists. For one, they are less available for study except in institutional settings. Ambulatory-based clinical trials are extremely difficult to field among the oldest old though some studies are now appearing. In addition, multiple coexisting diseases, both physical and psychiatric, often preclude the study of pure forms of psychiatric disorders, the staple of clinical trials. Though function varies widely among the oldest old, once people reach this age they frequently experience serious medical and/or psychiatry illness along with physical and social impairments which coalesce and cascade, often resulting in the condition described by geriatricians as frailty.[45, 46]

As the adverse physical and psychiatric consequences of age impinge upon the oldest old, the end result of this downward spiral is frailty and failure to thrive. Some have suggested that, after the age of 85, nearly half of all elders living in the community are frail despite their apparent functional well being.[47, 48] The manifestation of frailty most agreed upon is a constellation of weight loss, weakness, fatigue, inactivity, decreased food intake, confusion, memory impairment and depression. As can be seen, the two conditions described above— depression and Alzheimer's disease, conditions where psychiatry has made considerable advances in recent years among the elderly— may converge into a syndrome about which psychiatrists are especially frustrated in providing care.

Therefore psychiatrists might take a lesson from their geriatric colleagues and recognize that syndromes such as frailty may be critical to formulating appropriate care for the oldest old, the most vulnerable of the elderly. Comprehensive, interdisciplinary assessment and therapy, which are most applicable to the frail among the oldest old, was the cornerstone of the treatment of psychiatric disorders during the 1970s.[49, 50] Perhaps one of the major challenges for psychiatry during the next two decades is to translate the remarkable new findings regarding the psychopathology and treatment of depression and Alzheimer's disease in late life to the more complex comorbid conditions which find their final common pathway in frailty. In other words, the time has come for geriatric psychiatry to rejoin geriatric medicine so that we may recapture our roots and deliver optimal care to the oldest old as well as other persons 65 and older.

## References

1. Blazer, D. Geriatric psychiatry matures: advantages and problems as the psychiatry of old age grows older. *Current Opinion in Pyschiatr* 1998, 11: 401-403.

2. Blazer, D. Psychiatry and the oldest old. *Am J Psychiatr* 2000, 157: 1915-1924.

3. Older Americans 2000: Key Indicators of Well-being. Washington, DC: Federal Interagency Forum on Aging-Related Statistics, 2000.

4. Suzman, R. Oldest Old. In: Maddox, G., ed. Encyclopedia of Aging. New York: Springer, 1995: 712-715.

5. Schneider, L., Reynolds, C., Lebowitz, B., Friedhoff, A. Diagnosis and Treatment of Depression in Late Life. Washington, DC: American Psychiatric Press, 1994.

6. Evans, D., Funkenstein, H., Albert, M., *et al*: Prevalence of Alzheimer's disease in a community population of older persons: Higher than previously reported. *JAMA* 1989, 262: 2551-2556.

7. Reynolds, C., Frank, E., Perel, J., Imber, S., Cornes, C., Miller, M., Mazumdar, S., Houck, R., Dew, M., Stac, J., Pollock, B., Kupfer, D.: Nortriptyline and interpersonal psychotherapy as maintenance therapies for recurrent major depression: A randomized controlled trial in patients older than 59 years. *JAMA* 1999, 281: 39-45.

8. Kaufer, D., Cummings, J.: Neuropsychiatric aspects of Alzheimer's disease: the cholinergic hypothesis revisited. *Neurology* 1996, 47: 871-875.

9. Bartels, S., Colenda, C.: Mental health services for Alzheimer's disease: current trends in reimbursement, public policy, and the future under managed care. *Am J Geriatr Psychiatry* 1998, 6: 85-100.

10. Styron, W. Darkness Visible: A Memoir of Madness. New York: Random House, 1990.

11. Blazer, D.G., Kessler, R.C., McGonagle, K.A., Swartz, M.S.: The prevalence and distribution of major depression in the National Comorbidity Survey. *Am J Psychiatry* 1994, 151: 979-986.

12. Blazer, D., Burchett, B., Service, C., George, L: The association of age and depression among the elderly: An epidemiologic exploration. *J Geron Med Sci* 1991, 46: M210-215.

13. Hybles, C., Blazer, D., Pieper, C.: Toward a threshold for subthreshold depression: An analysis of correlates of depression by severity of symptoms using data from an elderly community survey. *Gerontologist* 2001, 41: 357-365.

14. Blazer, D. Depression in Late Life. St. Louis, MO: CV. Mosby and Company, 1994.

15. Bruce, M., Leaf, P.: Psychiatric disorders and 15-month mortality in a community sample of older adults. *Am J Pub Health* 1989, 79: 727-730.

16. Henderson, A., Korten, A., Jacomb, P., Mckinnon, A., Jorm, A., Christensen, H., Rodgers, B.: The course of depression in the elderly: a longitudinal community based study in Australia. *Psychol Med* 1997, 27: 119-129.

17. Takeida, K., Nishi, M., Miyake, H.: Zung's deprssion scale as a predictor of death in elderly people: a cohort study in Hokkaido, Japan. *J Epidemiol* 1999, 9: 240-244.

18. Koenig, H., Meador, K., Cohen, H., DG B: Depression in elderly hospitalized patients with medical illness. *Arch Intern Med* 1988, 148: 1929-1936.

19. Massie, J., Holland, J.: Depression and the cancer patient. *J Clin Psychiatr* 1990; 51 (suppl. 7): 12-17.

20. Reifler, B., Larson, E., Henley, R.: Coexistence of cognitive impairment and depression in geriatric outpatients. *Am J Psychiatr* 1982, 139: 623-626.

21. Hays, J., Saunders, W., Flint, E., Kaplan, B., Blazer, D.: Depression and social support as risk factors for functional disability in late life. *Aging Mental Health* 1997, 3: 209-220.

22. Inouye, S., Peduzzi, P., Robison, J., Hughes, J., Horwitz, R., Concato, J.: Importance of functional measures in predicting mortality among older adults. *JAMA* 1998, 279: 1187-1193.

23. Salive, M., Blazer, D : Depression and smoking cessation in older adults: a longitudinal study. *J Am Geriatr Soc* 1993, 41: 1313-1316.

24. Blazer, D.: Impact of late-life depression on the social network. *Am J Psychiatr* 1983, 140: 162-166.

25. Weissman, M., Bruce, M., Leaf, P., Florio, L., Holzer III, C. Affective Disorders. In: Regier, D.A., Robins, L.N., eds. Psychiatric Disorders in America. New York: The Free Press, 1991: 53-80.

26. Schoenfeld, D., Malmrose, L., Blazer, D., Gold, D., Seeman, T.: Self-rated health and mortality in the high-functioning elderly - A closer look at healthy individuals: MacArthur Field Study of Successful Aging. *J Gerontol Med Sci* 1994, 49: 109-M115.

27. Blazer, D.: Social support and mortality in an elderly community population. *Am J Epidemiol* 1982, 115: 684-694.

28. Unutzer, J., Patrick, D., Simon, G., Grembowski, D., Walker, E., Rutter, C., Katon, W.: Depressive symptoms and the cost of health services in HMO patients 65+ years and older. *JAMA* 1997; 277: 1618-1623.

29. Blazer, D., Hybels, C., Simonsick, E., Hanlon, J.: Marked differences in antidepressant use by race in an elderly community sample: 1986-1996. *Am J Psychiatr* 2000; 157: 1089-1094.

30. Krishnan, K., Hays, J., Blazer, D.: MRI-defined vascular depression. *Am J Psychiatr* 1997; 154:497-501.

31. Alexopoulas, G.: New concepts for prevention and treatment of late life depression. *Am J Psychiatr* 2001; 158:835-838.

32. Salzman, C. Pharmacological treatment of depression in elderly patients. In: Schneider, L., Reynolds, C., Lebowitz, B., Friedhoff, A., eds. Diagnosis and Treatment of Depression in Late Life. Washington, DC: American Psychiatric Press, 1994: 181-244.

33. Salzman, C. Psychopharmacologic therapy for late life depression: National Depression and Manic Depressive Association, 2001.

34. Small, G., Rabins, P., Barry, P.: Diagnosis and treatment of Alzheimer's Disease and related disorders: Consensus statement of the American Association of Geriatric Psychiatry, the Alzheimer's Association and the American Geriatric Society. *JAMA* 1997, 278: 1865-1870.

35. Tomlinson, E., Blessed, G., Roth, M.: Observations on the brains of demented old people. *J Neurol Sci* 1970, 11: 205-242.

36. Roses, A.: Apolipoprotein E affects the rate of Alzheimer disease expression: ß-amyloid burden is a secondary consequence dependent on APOE genotype and duration of disease. *J Neuropathol Exp Neurol* 1994, 53: 429-437.

37. Marx, J.: Bad for the heart, bad for the mind. *Science* 2001, 294: 508-509.

38. Saunders, A., Schmader, K., Breitner, J.: Apolipoprotein, E. epsilon 4 allele distributions in late-onset Alzheimer's disease and in other amyloid forming diseases. *Lancet* 1993, 342: 710-711.

39. Jick, H., Zornberg, G., Jick, S., Seshadri, S., Drachman, D.: Statins and the risk of dementia. *Lancet* 2000, 356: 1627-1631.

40. Fassbender, K., Simons, M., Bergman, C., Stroick, M., Lutjohann, D., Keller, P., Runz, H., Kuhl, S., Bersch, T., von Gergmann, K., Hennerici, M., Beyreuther, K., Hartman, T.: Simvastatin strongly reduces levels of Alzheimer's disease beta-amyloid peptides Abeta 42 and Abeta 40 in vitro and in vivo. *Proc Nat Acad Sci* 2001, 98: 5371-5373.

41. Katz, I., Jeste D, Mintzer J, Clyde C: Comparison of risperidone and placebo for psychoses and behavioral disturbances with dementia: A randomized double-blind trial. Risperidone Study Group. *J Clin Psychiatr* 1999, 60: 107-115.

42. Jeste, D., Alexopoulas, G., Bartels, S., Cummings, J., Gallo, J., Gottlieb, G., Halpain, M., Palmer, B., Patterson, T., Reynolds, C., Lebowitz, B.: Consensus statement on the upcoming crisis in geriatric mental healh care: Research agenda for the next 2 decades. *Arch Gen Psychiatry* 1999, 56: 848-853.

43. Callahan, C., Nienaber, N., Hendrie, H., Tierney, W.: Depression of elderly outpatients: primary care physicians attitudes and practice patterns. *J Gen Intern Med* 1992, 7: 26-31.

44. Callahan, C., Hendrie, H., Tierney, W.: Documentation and evaluation of cognitive impairment in elderly primary care patients. *Ann Intern Med* 1995, 122: 422-429.

45. Fried, L., Ettinger, W., Lind, B., Newman, A., Gardin, J.: Physical disability in older adults: a physiological approach. *J Clin Epidemiol* 1994, 47: 747-760

46. Fried, L. Frailty. In: Hazzard W, Bierman E, Blass J, Ettinger Jr. W, Halter J, eds. Principles of Geriatric Medicine and Gerontology. New York: McGraw Hill, 1994: 1149-1156.

47. Fried, L., Walston, J.. Frailty and failure to thrive. In: Hazzard, W., Blass, J., Ettinger, W., Halter, J., Ouslander, J., eds. Principles of Geriatric Medicine and Gerontology. New York: McGraw Hill, 1999: 1387-1402.

48. Verdery, R: Failure to thrive in older persons. *J Am Geriatr Soc* 1996, 44: 465-466.

49. Blazer, D., Maddox, G. Developing Geriatric Sevices in a Community Mental Health Center: A Case History of a University Based Affiliate Clinic. Durham, North Carolina: Duke University Center for Aging and Human Development, 1977.

50. Butler, R., Lewis, M. Aging and Mental Health. St. Louis: Mosby, C.V. 1973.

## Discussion Highlights, Session III

### Children

— The acute problem of providing care for children with mental disorders needs to be addressed. In Massachusetts, a state with the highest concentration of child psychiatrists in the country and an enlightened populace, care is "abysmal" because of policy decisions that put the mental health component of Medicaid out to competitive bid by for-profit HMOs. As a result, access to care for children has declined, with half of the beds closed, children stuck on pediatric wards and residential care facilities closed. In California, HMOs make coverage decisions based on strict medical definitions, so don't cover such problems as learning disabilities. As a result, care for children has become a struggle based on HMO reimbursement decisions rather than a rational approach to meeting a child's needs. Consumer involvement helps, but a parent faced with an ill child is not necessarily a rational consumer, as demonstrated by the push to get coverage for an untested therapy, facilitated communication, for autism and mentally retarded children.

— History has constrained research that would help deal with children who have been directly or secondarily traumatized. The number of investigators dealing with the problems of children is small and those investigators have controlled what research is done through their service on grant review committees, effectively blocking and discouraging work by those outside of that group.

### New Roles to Pediatricians

— Since pediatricians are going to treat a large number of young patients with mental health problems, pediatric residents need training in psychopharmacology so they know how to evaluate their patients and to be sure they are on the proper medication. Though pediatricians want to learn, few experts in child psychiatry are available to teach them. "Guild" issues are a further barrier, since residents are used for service, not for training. Pediatricians need to be trained to judge who should be on medication, what should be dispensed and at what dose. The same type of training is needed for family practitioners, for studies show that 80% of ritalin is prescribed by family practitioners, not pediatricians or psychiatrists. Currently, there is a mismatch between good diagnosis and who gets the medication. It is easy to turn the drug into a demon when the real issue is training and appropriate medicine.

## Children and Adolescents

— Given the overwhelming number of problems confronting child psychiatry, some way must be found to increase the current short supply of both trained child psychiatrists and child psychiatric researchers.

— More attention to cross-cultural diagnosis may be important, since it is not clear whether problems like attention deficit disorder are environmentally dependent or whether this is a problem in China or in Europe.

— Anxiety and depression are especially difficult to diagnose in young children who are not good at expressing themselves. Behavior is easy to diagnose by observation; anxiety and depression, which are internal states, are not.

— The lack of application of what is known about the care and well being of children is a constant challenge. When children have problems, it is important also to consider parents and siblings to see if there are similar disorders. Since ritalin is not going to help a child if the father is an alcoholic and the mother is depressed, it is important to treat the parents as well as the child. Often parents of child patients become the adult patients. Implementing that kind of logic does not demand more research, but it does suggest a new look at the goals of disciplines if professional limitations mean that a child psychiatrist does not deal with parents.

— Incremental changes will not solve current problems in child psychiatry. Instead key competencies should be identified and then taught to both pediatric and adult psychiatrists, eliminating the idea that advocacy for one member of a family makes it impossible to treat others.

— The emotional climate and child rearing practices of parents need to be considered, especially with children who have parents with a major mental disorder. Studies have shown clear patterns of systematic effects on the children. The most damaging are on children raised by parents who are depressed. Since depression is the most prevalent major disorder, this is a significant finding yet a psychiatrist with an adult patient being treated for depression may not even know whether that patient has children.

Based on this new information, several clinics and children's hospitals have developed intervention programs for the children of depressed adults to test whether care and treatment of the parent will prevent the occurrence of mental illness in the child.

— Expertise to guide the judiciary system on the use of psychopharmaceuticals in children is missing. The assumption is made that children have been appropriately diagnosed and treated but, in reality, restrictions on providing psychiatric services for children call that assumption into question. In Massachusetts, for instance,the ability to treat children is so restricted that the response to a child in crisis often is to add another medication, since there is not enough time to remove a medication or adjust dosages in a protected environment.

— A number of reports indicate substantial growth in the use of psychopharmaceuticals in young children. One paper from Michigan documented the use of prescription psychotropic medications in 80 Medicaid children under the age of two; 70% of them received more than one medication and less than 40% received psychological treatment. Such studies raise concerns about potential misuse of medications, use by individuals not qualified to make a diagnosis, and, because of the perceived cost of behavioral treatment, complete neglect of family and behavioral interventions.

— The field needs to stop sending the message that everything can be treated with medications. It is important to understand the limitations of pharmacology and to ask if other treatments might have meant fewer or no medications. With children, there is a range of complementary, behavioral and school-based therapies that are not applied.

— The gap between new information coming from research in the neurosciences and the treatment of children is huge, and growing. Adult psychiatrists need to understand this information and learn about the treatment of children, since all disorders except Alzheimer's disease and dementia begin early. All medical and other health professional students should have mandated courses on mental disorders in children, as should psychologists, social workers and school counselors.

— School clinics ought to be "islands of hope in a sea of despair," yet few do their work effectively. A study of school based clinics in several schools in poor areas showed about half of the children do not come regularly, 100% of the professionals have no exposure to "evidence-based anything," turnover among social workers is rapid because of poor working conditions, and clinics close abruptly because they run out of funds. When half of the children do not come to school, school psychologists should stop testing and try to find what needs to be done to get them back into school.

— Many children suffer because of continued exposure to violence. Teachers need to know how to recognize when a child has a problem but, because of the teacher shortage, few have the necessary training. Of the 35,000 teachers in the Los Angeles schools, 25% are not trained, a problem with a population where 21% have a diagnosable mental disorder. Many teachers who see these problems every day do not have the information they need to bring it to professional attention. As a result, problems are hidden in plain sight.

— The shift from psychodynamic to evidence-based psychotherapy is a cognitive shift, but school clinics involve shifts of resources and a reallocation of dollars and expertise to inner-city schools. This is not a dichotomy between public health or population-based approaches care, and individual care but between the haves and have nots.

— The push by many groups to add qualifications for everything from addiction medicine to the psychiatric care of the mentally ill and psychsomatic medicine has hidden costs. Not only does it contribute to fragmentation of the field, but it affects training programs, curriculum, and the ability to develop fellowship programs. It is not clear how to add experience in therapies and psychopharmacology, or understanding how to add care for elderly people with medical illnesses into already crowded residency programs or into the single hour too many students have for training in these areas.

— Attention needs to be paid to the damaging effects of the media, especially television, on children and families and on their expectations. This is especially true of the media attentiion provided for violence, abuse, and sexuality

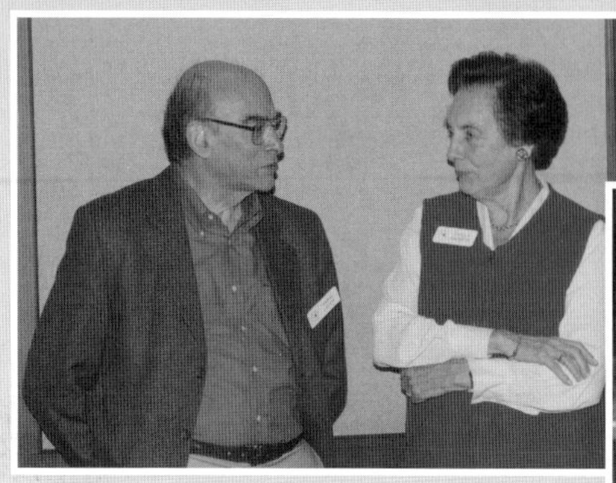

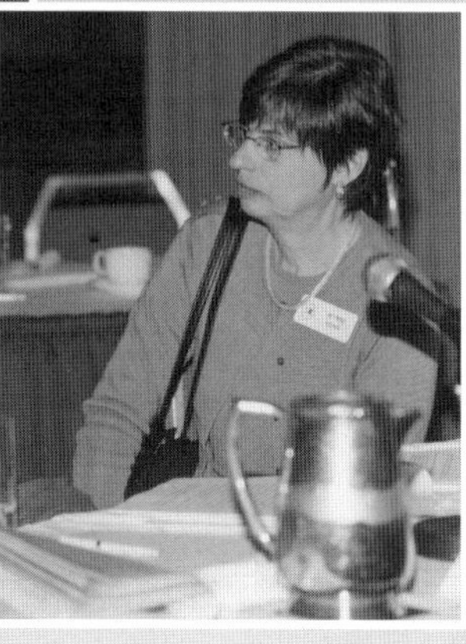

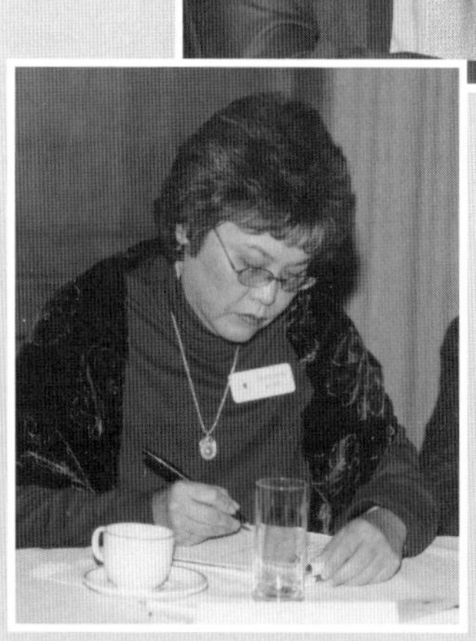

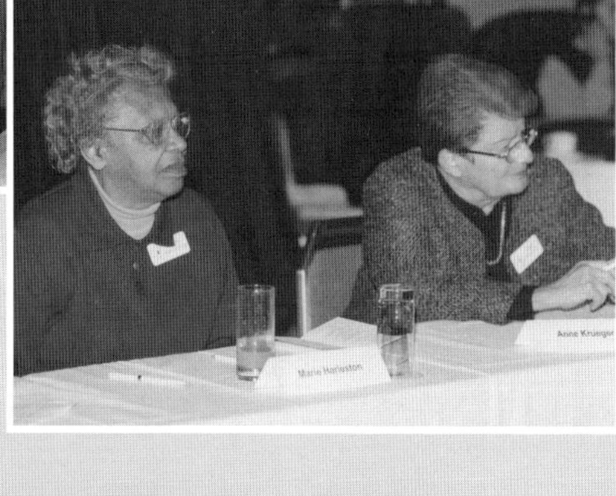

Marie Harleston

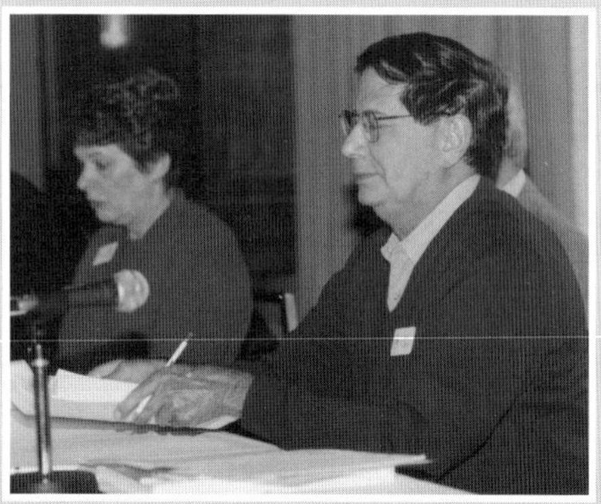

# Session IV

## Disparities in Mental Disorders

*The fact of significant, systematic and continuing disparities in health and mental health outcomes has been known for many decades. These gaps are most prominent among the poor, and among racial and ethnic minority groups. The session opened with a discussion of poverty and mental health because of the very strong linkage of poverty with racial and ethnic minority status. This enabled the participants to sort out the underlying poverty factors such as inadequacy of personal and community resources to meet basic needs, the high stress of living in neighborhoods with drugs, violence and poor schools. This was followed by a report of the factors specific to Blacks that included, recommended treatment approaches that are culturally sensitive along with representing high quality, evidence-based care and promising lines of needed clinical research. A discussion of special issues for Hispanic populations was then presented.*

## Poverty and Mental Illness: Educating Health Professionals to Meet New Needs

**Paula Allen-Meares,**
**Dean, Norma Radin Collegiate Professor of Social Work**
**Co-Principal Investigator, NIMH Center on Poverty, Risk, and Mental Health, University of Michigan School of Social Work**

### Introduction

I want to thank Drs. Osborn and Hamburg, and the Foundation's Board of Directors for inviting me to be a part of the Macy Conference on Modern Psychiatry and to help facilitate the discussion regarding disparities in mental disorders. I am delighted to join you and am honored to participate in this important discussion regarding the challenges and opportunities we face in training the next generation of mental and other health professionals to meet changing needs in our society as we face the gap between the extraordinary pace of research advances, and the factors that challenge their translation into our communities. I am particularly pleased to respond to your request by focusing my remarks on the links between poverty and mental disorders, as we discuss disease determinants that undermine availability of services for specific components of our society. I am also very pleased to comment on the role of the University of Michigan School of Social Work's NIMH Center on Poverty, Risk, and Mental Health social work as an example of a new paradigm for delivery of mental health and other health care services to the most underserved elements of our communities, particularly as research and training. Social workers now represent the dominant profession providing services for individuals with mental illness and often find themselves working with and on behalf of the economically needy. It serves us well to remind ourselves of Mrs. Kate Macy Ladd's words in 1930 when she endowed the Macy Foundation, noting that "health is more than freedom from sickness."

We have emerged from the Decade of the Brain into an entirely new century and new millennium with an unparalleled wealth of research advances, but at the same time, we must recognize that the rapid pace of scientific discovery has dwarfed the ability of all mental and other health professionals to develop effective educational programs or models to deliver services. Mental health and other health professionals face entirely new challenges. Recent changes in psychopharmacology and rehabilitative technologies have created new modalities of treatment — but disparities in access to these treatments within underrepresented segments of our population can limit their efficacy. Significant determinants — including poverty, racism, inequality, health problems, stress, and trauma, among others — contribute to the incidence and severity of mental health disorders, particularly in our most underserved communities. Despite the staggering breadth of investigative advances that have occurred in biomedical research advances, we are severely compromised in our efforts to translate this knowledge into effective and accessible delivery of preventive and therapeutic treatments and to train mental health professionals in the most timely and informed ways. Nowhere is this more apparent than in impoverished segments of our society.

In order to discuss disparities in mental disorders and to recommend training modalities to best address them, these areas will be discussed:

A. poverty as a determinant of mental health and other health disorders,

B. the interaction of poverty and mental health,

C. the influence of poverty on depression,

D. the effects of welfare reform on mental health,

E. the effects of poverty on the mental well-being and development of children and youth,

F. racism and inequality as risk factors for mental health,

G. collaborative solutions including life sciences initiatives and evidence-based research interventions that hold promise for the mental health profession, and

H. ways in which we can create a new paradigm for mental health professional education.

## POVERTY AS A DETERMINANT OF MENTAL HEALTH DISORDERS

### Key Issues Regarding Poverty

To address the critical gaps between our wealth of information and actual service delivery to those who would benefit most, we need to understand key issues regarding poverty. A careful look at our recent past reveals growing gaps in family incomes and living conditions that have created lasting disparities between high-income and low-income communities and between the majority population and racial and ethnic minorities. Despite a sustained period of unprecedented economic growth in the 1990s, the poverty rates among children, older youth, and families — especially single mother-headed families of color — actually remain higher than they were in the 1970s. The economic growth that we have experienced since the 1970s has been uneven and slow, differing dramatically from the "rising tide lifting all boats" that led to post-World War II economic prosperity, which was widely shared by the poor, middle class, and the rich, as well as by the less skilled and the skilled worker. Today, structural changes in the labor market since the early 1970s have prevented many less-educated workers from securing lasting employment that could lead to economic independence. Other factors, including decline in union membership, reductions in manufacturing employment, increased global competition, and the expansion of import and export sectors, all led to the lowering of wages for less-skilled workers. (Danziger, S. 2001). Computerization of the workplace also increased demand for skilled personnel and displaced less-skilled workers, especially welfare recipients. Welfare recipients and other impoverished members of our communities face more barriers to employment — they have less work experience, more child care responsibilities, and are more likely to experience gender or racial discrimination. (Danziger, S.K. *et al.* 2000). Recent statistics also demonstrate that we now are experiencing the biggest gap between the rich and the poor in our country's history, and that the United States has the largest impoverished poverty population of any industrialized nation.

## Interaction of Mental Health and Poverty

The interaction of mental health and poverty is an important area of focus. The stresses of low socioeconomic status may cause or exacerbate mental health problems, and mental illness may lead to lower socioeconomic status by interfering with the ability to improve one's education or income (Jayakody, Danziger & Pollack, 1999). Individuals in disadvantaged communities can be trapped in deteriorating neighborhoods, dysfunctional families, dangerous schools, and negative stereotypes. Thus, low socioeconomic status (SES) has been recognized as both a determinant and an outcome of mental disorders. Consequences of mental problems such as depression are markedly different for low-skilled workers in environments without significant health benefits. Depression among individuals with low SES frequently remains undetected or inadequately treated (Ford 1994). Barriers to employment — including low education level, little work experience, child care challenges, and transportation problems — also represent barriers to workers' mental health since they can determine whether a woman can find and keep a job (Siefert, *et al.*, 2000). Researchers analyzing data from the 1994 and 1995 National Household Survey of Drug Abuse, for example, found that in the year preceding the study, 19% of welfare recipients had experienced a psychiatric disorder. Because the study measured only four psychiatric disorders, it probably underestimated the prevalence of mental disorders among low-income individuals. The study also identified mental health problems as being more prevalent than substance abuse among low-income single mothers (Jayakody, Danziger, & Pollack, 1999). Other studies suggest that post-traumatic stress disorder and social phobia are also prevalent diagnoses among low-income single mothers (Grommet *et al.*,1998). Data from the National Comorbidity Study has demonstrated that 35% of low income women surveyed have either major depression, Post Traumatic Stress Disorder, general anxiety disorder, alcohol dependence, or drug dependence. (Bromet *et al.*, 1998). In addition, studies are being conducted to assess the prevalence of psychiatric disorders, physical disabilities and domestic violence among low income single mothers to identify interrelationships and to examine the links from these problems to unemployment and dependency (Siefert, *et al.*, 2000).

What we know from other empirical studies is that persons with schizophrenia experience low levels of employment and vocational functioning for many years after the onset of their illnesses (Cook & Razzano, 2000). Furthermore, follow-up studies of cohorts with schizophrenia have found that vocational rehabilitation interventions do not work as well for these individuals when compared with other psychiatric disorders. In one study, it was reported that a consistent but small minority (8-40%) of persons with schizophrenia manage to work (Cook & Razzano, 2000). It appears that people with this particular disorder have poor employment and vocational outcomes with compared to other disorders.

## The Influence of Poverty on Depression

Depression is one example of the intersection between poverty and mental health. Although biological, social, and demographic risk factors have been identified for depression, the mechanisms through which these risk factors do or do not lead to depression are not clear, and many risk factors are not modifiable. Worldwide epidemiological studies have established that depression occurs twice as often in women as in men and that a peak in first onset occurs in the child-bearing and child-rearing years (Culbertson, 1997). Other data have shown that mothers with several young children, single mothers, and mothers in poverty are at heightened risk of depression (Hobfoll *et al.*, 1995). Because women are over-represented among poor populations, and because poverty is a determinant of depression, the intersection between poverty and mental health becomes all the more apparent.

Poverty increases the likelihood of exposure to acute and chronic stressors associated with depression (such as exposure to violence, unemployment and low-wage work, limited opportunities, and poor health), and decreases access to material and emotional resources that help mitigate the impact of these stressors. Women of color are over-represented among low-income mothers and also face racial discrimination, suggested by recent research findings to be a key risk factor for mental health problems (Amaro, Russo, & Johnson 1987). Welfare recipients have considerably higher rates of depression than non-recipients. A case-controlled study of homeless and housed women receiving welfare found a 43% lifetime prevalence rate of major depression (Salomon, Bassuk, & Brooks 1996). As major depression can be recurring and become more severe with subsequent episodes, the public health consequences are obvious — particularly for individuals who live in situations which present few options for improvement. For these individuals, environmental factors beyond traditional risks may influence depression — and could represent factors that could be modified or perhaps eliminated.

## The Effects of Welfare Reform on Mental Health

Welfare reform, introduced in 1996, also affected impoverished individuals with mental problems. The reform law limited the number of years an individual can receive federal benefits, required employment as a condition of receiving benefits, and emphasized immediate work experience over training. These changes affected many recipients, especially those with psychiatric disorders. Individuals with substance abuse and mental health problems had limited ability to participate effectively in training programs or to leave welfare for work within specified times. Another issue affecting the intersection between poverty and mental health is the documented unmet need for mental health services. A one-year follow-up study of barriers to work among welfare mothers following welfare reform found the twelve-month prevalence of major depression to be 25%. The study also showed that mothers meeting diagnostic screening criteria for major depression were significantly less likely to make the transition from welfare to work than mothers not meeting the criteria (Danziger *et al.*, 2000). It is also known that despite the high occurrence of mental health problems in impoverished communities, few individuals with these problems actually receive treatment. This is further exacerbated by the decline in Medicaid enrollment of welfare recipients, and results of surveys document that almost half of former recipients do not have health insurance after leaving welfare for work (Chavkin, Romero, & Wise 2000).

## Effects on the Well-being of Children and Youth

Poverty and inequality affect the well-being of children and families. Despite our unprecedented prosperity, more than one fifth of our nation's children are being raised in poverty. Although national welfare rolls dropped by more than 50% between 1993 and 2001, child poverty rates dropped only 17%. In New York alone, welfare caseloads declined by 30% but child poverty decreased by only 7%. In 1999, after nearly a decade of unprecedented economic growth, one in six American children — over 12 million children — lived in poverty, according to figures from the U.S. Census Bureau. The relationship between income and infant mortality has been well documented. Despite our wealth, the United States has neither the longest average life span nor the lowest infant mortality rate. The United States ranks first among industrialized countries in childhood death rates. The excess mortality is attributable to unintentional injuries and violence, many of which are caused by socioeconomic factors such as poor housing and dangerous neighborhoods. Chronic health conditions are a major risk factor for school failure and placement in special education classes, and food insecurity and hunger represent substantial problems for impoverished children, as well. In addition, parents struggling with poverty frequently have poor nurturing relationships with their infants, which often result in infant mental health problems. Without intervention, these children can grow up troubled within a cycle of challenges. Effective parenting is further hampered by the over-representation of poorly educated people and people with mental illness among poor populations. Poor families are much more likely to have substantiated cases of child maltreatment, particularly child neglect, than families with adequate incomes. Reports of child maltreatment continue to be made in record numbers, now over 3 million per year. The escalating problem of child abuse and neglect has also led to a crisis in the foster care system.

Developmental outcomes are less positive in offspring of parents with mental illness. A meta— analysis of multiple research studies has illustrated negative consequences of parental depression on children and adolescents (Oyserman & Allen-Meares, in production). As many as 50% of the offspring of these parents will experience a serious affective disorder, and therefore face a significantly greater risk of mental illness than children of non-depressed parents (Beardslee and Wheelock, 1994). Longitudinal studies have also documented long-term consequences, and have demonstrated the occurrence of higher rates of major depression, phobias, panic disorder, and alcohol dependence in offspring of affectively ill parents. (Weissman *et al.* 1997).

A number of studies have also documented linkages between community and neighborhood conditions and child and adolescent well-being and developmental outcomes (Coulton, Korbin, & Su, 1996). Several studies have developed neighborhood measures to investigate the influences of risk factors and social interaction as determinants of externalizing and internalizing behavior patterns among disadvantaged youth (Leventhal & Brooks-Gunn, 2000). Recent research has also illustrated that persistent poverty vs. transitory poverty has more significant effects on school achievement and socioeconomic function (McLoyd, 1998).

### Racial and Ethnic Inequality as Risk Factors for Mental Illnesses

Poverty alone does not account for pronounced racial disparities in almost all indicators of well-being in the United States. Racism and ethnic inequality are pervasive adverse influences, as well. As a number of scholars have noted, institutionalized racism and discrimination can restrict socioeconomic mobility and lead to low socioeconomic status and exposure to poor living conditions (Williams *et al* 1997). Some researchers have linked subjective experiences of discriminatory treatment to higher rates of mental health and health problems, which in turn affect social, occupational, and family functioning (Amaro, Russo, & Johnson 1987). Although African American mental illness rates are overall comparable to those of whites, they are accompanied by more experiences of racial discrimination associated with psychological distress and depression (Kessler, Mickelson, & Williams 1999).

Every mental health professional whom we train and with whom we collaborate should be concerned about poverty and inequality, because these factors make equality of opportunity and access to necessary and appropriate services harder to attain. The children of the poor— especially children of color— receive lower quality education and health care, and live in more dangerous communities. Older youth in these circumstances face challenges in their ability to afford or complete career training or higher education. Single mothers who are racial and ethnic minorities are not only at higher risk of poverty, but their opportunities are constrained by the effects of historical and contemporary discrimination. Although we have never been wealthier as a nation, millions of families still have difficulty making ends meet, and their access to adequate preventive care treatment is compromised. Poverty and inequality in earnings and in family income are higher today than they were three decades ago. Millions of less skilled workers and former welfare recipients have significant difficulty earning enough to support their families, despite a low unemployment rate nationwide. In a society increasingly defined by high-tech opportunities, many high school dropouts, welfare recipients, and even high school graduates encounter significant difficulty obtaining stable employment that will allow them to earn enough to escape the confines of poverty. The reduced demand for less-skilled workers has been accompanied by an increase in economic hardship and a sustained level of poverty despite tight labor markets. Contrary to our nation's commitment to equality of opportunity, our country provides a far less effective safety net than do other major industrialized nations.

## Collaborative Solutions

In order to address these multiple, but related, determinants of health disparities, we need to work together to reverse these trends. Social work is the leading health-related profession with an explicit commitment to oppressed and underserved groups. The profession's roots trace back to the mid-nineteenth century. Over one hundred years later, many benefits and social institutions on which so many individuals rely— child labor laws, health and housing for the urban poor, maternal and child health services, and Social Security— owe their existence, in part, to the efforts of social workers to address social injustice.

Bench and Trench Partnerships. Some institutions, including the University of Michigan, have invested in far-reaching plans targeting the life sciences. It is critical that disciplines and professions beyond those actively engaged in basic bench research become active partners in these initiatives in order to ensure translation of research into practice— and to facilitate effective service delivery of new modalities of care in our communities, including the most disenfranchised segments of our society. Our school has partnered in the University of Michigan's Life Sciences Initiative in a unique plan for research and instructional investment addressing the intersection between social environment and health.

The consideration of ethics, the inclusion of disadvantaged populations in study groups, the recognition of socioeconomic barriers to access new developments in health and mental health care , and the impact of our social environment on well-being are all key topics for health and mental health professionals to address collaboratively. Many risk factors for disease that have been identified are global and not readily modified for specific populations — particularly the more vulnerable and underserved segments of our society. The vast amount of knowledge generated by research in genetics has raised an equally vast volume of issues and questions regarding the use of this information and access to it. Many of these issues may be of particular concern to individuals from diverse or disadvantaged communities who may not be familiar with this area of research or whose prior exclusion from research studies may have contributed to disparities in the diagnostic and treatment options available to members of these groups. Similarly, inclusion of members of these populations in earlier studies may have increased stigmatization or have determined discrimination in health insurance, health care, or employment. There is a need to ensure effectively designed, interdisciplinary research that can help resolve and reduce unequal participation of minority populations in clinical research trials. In addition, there is a need to increase the volume of minority researchers involved in this work, and a corresponding need to recognize this in our training programs, in order to develop effective pipelines for career development. The involvement of social workers in genetic services research can increase the likelihood of meaningful findings affecting adoption policy and the use of genetic information in adoption procedures; access to testing services for underserved and disadvantaged populations; the use of genetic information in the school setting; and identification of gaps in genetic services. These initiatives are compatible with newly defined research objectives at NIH, which promote research projects which examine: issues raised by the integration of genetic technologies and information into health care and public health activities; the ways in which new knowledge may interact with a variety of perspectives; and the influences of socioeconomic factors, gender, race, ethnicity, and culture on the use and interpretation of genetics information, the utilization of genetic services, and the development of policy.

Mental health represents another potential area for collaboration with the life sciences. Long-term psychiatric disorders (such as schizophrenia, bipolar disorder, major affective disorder, and obsessive-compulsive disorder) may occur in small percentages of our population, but affect entire families in the course of treatment and in access to care. Genetic factors appear to be relevant in individual predisposition to such disorders, but environmental factors are required for expression of these illnesses, and many socioeconomic factors may influence the course and success of treatments. Although social workers represent the dominant professional service providers to individuals with serious mental illnesses, most definitive research to date has been conducted by other health professionals. As a result, there are major limitations to interpretation and meaning in terms of dependent and independent variables selected for study, which may not be the most reliable indicators of longer-term outcomes. Social work and psychology researchers can contribute selection of more appropriate predictor variables — such as maternal or early childhood stress.

The University of Michigan School of Social Work's NIMH Center on Poverty, Risk, & Mental Health. (see Figure 1) The Center on Poverty, Risk, and Mental Health represents a unique intellectual resource at our School that has enhanced our understanding of poverty and mental health as co-determinants through innovative, interdisciplinary evidence-based research projects. The Center is an interdisciplinary unit that involves campuswide collaborators from the School of Social Work; the School of Public Health; the Ford School of Public Policy; the Medical School; the Department of Psychiatry; the College of Literature, Science & Arts; the Institute for Social Research; the Center for Human Growth and Development; and the Psychology and Political Science Departments. The Center's research focuses on the psychiatric epidemiology and descriptive studies of low-income single mothers, preventive interventions, and mental health services for the poor. Various studies under its auspices have proven to be particularly timely, having been initiated at the advent of welfare reform, and having led to the development of a unique database measuring the full range of barriers to employment of welfare mothers and to a variety of preventive interventions and mental health services. These include the Women's Employment Study and Mothers' Well-Being Study databases, which contain critical information regarding important barriers in the transition from welfare-to-work. These data have led to recommendations that

**FIGURE 1**

**Social Work Research Development Center**
**Poverty, Risk and Mental Health**
**Core Research Areas and Collaborative Relationships**

Center for Human Growth and Development
RESEARCH DEVELOPMENT CENTER
SCHOOL OF SOCIAL WORK
ADMINISTRATION AND RESEARCH SUPPORT
• Administration
• Governance Advisory Board
• Research Seminar on Poverty, Risk and Mental Health
CORE RESEARCH AREAS
• Epidemiological Research on Social Class and Mental Illness
• Developmental Research on Effects of High-Risk Environments on Children
• Preventive Interventions: Organizational Readiness and Needs Assessment in Welfare-to-Work Programs
• Service Research
Institute for Social Research
Survey Research Center
Research and Training Program on Poverty, the Underclass, and Public Policy
Michigan Program on Poverty and Social Welfare Policy
Michigan Prevention Research Center
Department of Psychiatry Medical School
Institute for Research on Women and Gender
Program on Psychological Factors in Mental Health and Illness
African American Mental Health Research center

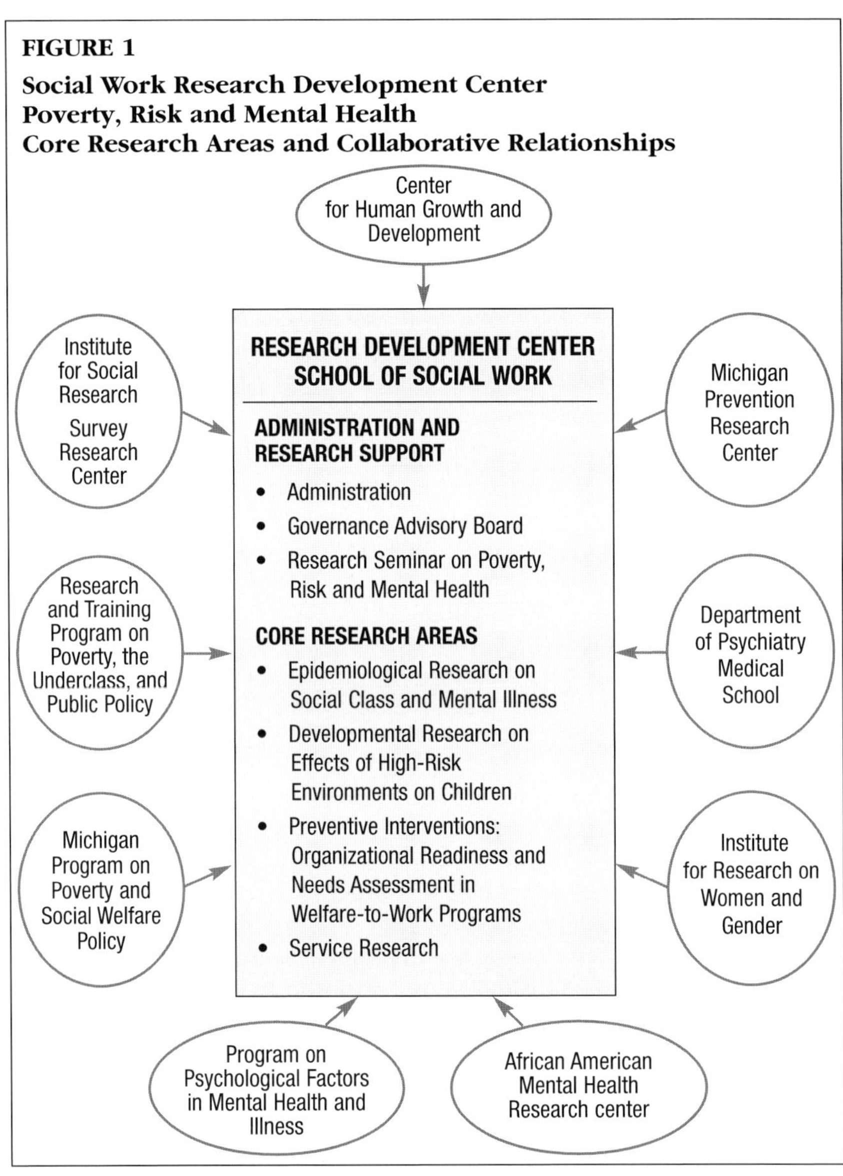

enable welfare applicants to be screened for mental illness and referred for treatment to improve upon current welfare to work programs which do not perform testing or screening, and which assume that all applicants are somehow employable. These longitudinal studies have demonstrated that the ability of women on welfare to work is compromised by a range of family, physical, and mental health barriers (Corcoran, M., Danziger, S.K., Kalil, A., & Seefeldt, K., 2000). They also have gathered important data on low-income single mothers who, as a group, have been underrepresented in previous studies of psychiatric problems, physical disabilities, and domestic violence. Despite the established association between depression and welfare reliance among single mothers, prior studies on other disorders had not recognized welfare recipients as a distinct subject population.

Another Center intervention study is a Substance Abuse and Welfare Reform project focusing on the relationship between substance abuse, mental health problems, welfare receipt, and employment. The study's data should enhance our understanding of the relationship between these problems and developing treatment and other services to address them (Jayakody *et al.*, 2000). Another study addresses Food Insecurity, Mental Health, and Welfare Reform. It has established demographic profiles of welfare recipients who experience food insecurity, changes in rate of food insecurity over time, and the relation of food insecurity to mental health and child development (Siefert *et al.*, 2001). Data from this project will be essential to the planning and evaluation of nutrition programs and policy development. The Michigan Family Study is another longitudinal study associated with the Center and the University's Department of Pediatrics, which has focused on stages of infant development — a neglected area in child mental health research. The study has examined infant mental health risk factors associated with poverty, including economic hardship, adverse neighborhood conditions, stress, and poor parental mental health. The study's goal is to identify target behaviors that could lead to the development of a model of prevention that could be applied to infants at greatest risk. This study fills a gap in research knowledge which could expand services for infants in community clinics and pediatric practices.

The Center has also enhanced the development of mental health services research. Center research includes a cost-benefit analysis of supported education, providing strategic planning and technical assistance for communities. Another project addresses contextual risk and resilience in African American adolescents. Another example of Center research is an intervention benefit/cost analysis study to Reduce Recurrent Homelessness Among Severely Mentally Ill Men. The intervention has demonstrated that treatment leads to lower costs and reduced homelessness by enabling more independent living, decreased use of mental health care services, and reduced shelter use. Social work researchers are also developing ways to affect the documented link between early mental illness onset and negative educational outcomes.

## Preparing the Next Generation of Health Professionals

The students we are training will all need to be better informed about the diverse populations to whom health and mental health care are delivered. The mental health professionals of tomorrow are likely to be confronted with issues regarding prevention and at-risk populations, for example, and will need to be able to assess how genetic factors affect the lives of vulnerable families, individuals, and communities. Together, we all share an obligation to understand the ethical, legal, and social implications surrounding the application of new technology and the availability of new information; we also share a responsibility to translate research findings into practice applications. In training the next generation of health professionals, we must understand the influence of environmental contributors to the onset, course, and outcome of health and mental health problems, such as poverty and discrimination; the modification or elimination of risk factors related to poverty and social inequality; the influence of poverty, race, ethnicity, and culture on access to and use of health information and services; and the social implications of integrating new technology and information into clinical and non-clinical settings for those populations which are most vulnerable to exploitation or discrimination.

We cannot move forward as professionals or as members of society without collaboration beyond traditional disciplines. Future research funding opportunities will increasingly demand this, and our training programs for health and mental health professionals will be less effective without this. This must be a fundamental element in the training we offer. Postdoctoral opportunities such as those funded by the Ford Foundation in our School's Center on Poverty, Risk, and Mental Health, provide a successful example of an interdisciplinary, collaborative training model. We must include consideration of socioeconomic determinants and circumstances that can influence health care problems, and include this as a fundamental aspect of our training. We must recognize the changing demographics of our population, including increases in life expectancy that are unlikely to be accompanied by continued good health, especially among the disadvantaged. Therefore, we need to optimize health maintenance and eliminate barriers, and include these as fundamental aspects of our training. In addition, we have to recognize that our superb advances in health care technology are useless if services are not widely available — and we therefore must ensure that access to effective health care is ensured for all segments of our population, and underscore that within our training. Finally, we have to recognize the diversity of our population and the cultural contexts of illness — and include these considerations as fundamental parts of our training.

The educational preparation of health/mental health professionals and researchers must emphasize the translation of research into practice. Two recent NIMH reports, *Bridging Science & Service (1999)* and *Translating Behavioral Science Into Action* (2000), focus on this issue. For example, psychopharmacology treatments are developed in controlled settings: How do we implement them in the real world, (especially the world of individuals who already have multiple demands and stressors)? One would also need to address behavior change — which requires an understanding of the person, medication regimens as prescribed, follow-through on treatments, and necessary lifestyle changes.

Partnerships with communities will be a fundamental aspect of our research, interventions, and training programs. For effective collaborations, we must build trust with communities in which we collect research data. In many situations, there is an enormous lack of trust and uncertainty about the application of data and value to the community with "hit and run" research projects. In all too many instances, there are perceptions that many academic researchers enter communities, collect research data, and then leave without returning to the community or helping solve the problems they study. Innovations at places like the University of Michigan are addressing these problems by establishing joint consortia of community agencies and academic researchers to help develop ways to renew trust and create reciprocal partnerships.

We live in a time where well-being is viewed as a national priority, at a time when researchers recognize the need to promote health prevention and well-being over an exclusive focus on acute health care; at a time when providers should attend to management of chronic conditions, rather than rely on development of future cures; and at a time when the pace of discovery outstrips our ability to always deliver services to those who need them the most. In an era of managed care when fewer patients are hospitalized and the ones who are hospitalized are more acutely ill, we increasingly need a team approach as we try to prevent health problems from recurring or occurring at all. It is precisely because some of the leading causes of death are chronic disorders where risk factors can be ameliorated that we need to work together to promote well-being, develop best practices, evaluate outcomes, and determine if our system provides the delivery of care to all who need it.

We have entered a new millenium where we have the opportunity and responsibility to redesign the way we train future health professionals. The Macy Foundation is helping lead the way by funding initiatives to improve health professional education, increase teamwork between different health disciplines, develop educational strategies to promote increased access to health care resources by underserved populations, and increase diversity among health care professionals. We can enhance these initiatives by creating a new training paradigm that fosters interdisciplinary teams of health professionals, encourages the translation of research findings to policy makers and practitioners, and ensures that advances in health care can be made available to the most vulnerable components of our society.

## References

Amaro, H., Russo, M.F., and Johnson, J. (1987). Family and work predictors of psychological well-being among Hispanic women professionals. *Psychology of Women Quarterly*, 11: 505-521.

Beardslee, W.R., and Wheelock, I. (1994). Children of parents with affective disorders: Empirical findings and clinical implications. In W. M. Reynolds & H.F. Johnston (Eds.), Handbook of Depression in Children and Adolescents (pp. 463-479). New York, NY: Plenum Press.

Bromet, E., Sonnega, A., and Kessler, R.C. (1998). Risk factors for DSM-III-R posttraumatic stress disorder: Findings from the National Comorbidity Survey. *American Journal of Epidemiology*, 147, 352-361.

Chavkin, W., Romero, D., and Wise, P.H. (2000). State welfare reform policies and declines in health insurance. *American Journal of Public Health*, 90: 900-908.

Cook, J., & Razzano, L. (2000). Vocational rehabilitation for persons with schizophrenia: Recent research and implications for practice. *Schizophrenia Bulletin*, 26: 87-103.

Corcoran, M., Danziger, S.K., Kalil, A., and Seefeldt, J. (2000). How welfare reform is affecting women's work. *Annual Review of Sociology*, 26: 241-269.

Coulton, C.J., Korbin, J.E., and Su, M. (1996). Measuring neighborhood context for young children in an urban area. *American Journal of Community Psychology*, 24: 5-32.

Culbertson, F.M. (1997). Depression and gender: An international review. *American Psychologist*, 52: 25-31.

Danziger, S. (2001). Welfare Reform Policy from Nixon to Clinton: What Role for Social Science? In D.C. Featherman & M.A. Vinovskis (Eds.) Social Science and Policy Making (pp. 137-164). Ann Arbor. MI: University of Michigan Press.

Danziger, S.K., Corcoran, M., Danziger, S., and Heflin, C. (2000). Work, income, and material hardship after welfare reform. *Journal of Consumer Affairs*, 34: 6-30.

Ford, D. (1994). Recognition and underrecognition of mental disorders in adult primary care. In J. Miranda, A. Hohmann, C. Attkisson, & D. Larson (Eds.), Mental Disorders in Primary Care (pp. 186-205). San Francisco: Jossey-Bass.

Hobfoll, S.E., Ritter, C., Lavin, J., Hulxizer, M.R., and Cameron, R.P. (1995). Depression prevalence and incidence among inner-city pregnant and postpartum women. *Journal of Consulting and Clinical Psychology*, 63, 445-453.

Jayakody, R., Danziger, S.K., and Pollack, H. (2000). Mental health problems, substance abuse and welfare reform. *Journal of Health Politics, Policy and Law*, 25: 623-665.

Jayakody, R. and Stauffer, D. (2000). Mental health problems among single mothers: implications for welfare reform. *Journal of Social Issues*, 56: 617-634.

McLoyd, V.C. (1998). Socioeconomic disadvantage and child development. *American Psychologist*, 53: 185-204.

National Institute of Mental Health. (1999). Bridging Science and Service (NIH Publication No. 99-4353). Washington, DC: U.S. Government Printing Office.

National Institute of Mental Health (2000). Translating Behavioral Science into Action. (NIH Publication No. 00-4699). Washington, DC: U.S. Government Printing Office.

Oyserman, D. and Allen-Meares, P. (in preparation). Offspring of Parents with Mental Illness: A Cluster Analysis of Developmental Outcomes.

Oyserman, D., Mowbray, C.T., Allen-Meares, P., & Firminger, K.B., (in press). Parenting among mothers with a serious mental illness. *American Journal of Orthopsychiatry.*

Salomon, A., Bassuk, S.S., and Brooks, M.G. (1996). Patterns of welfare use among poor and homeless women. *American Journal of Orthopsychiatry*, 66: 510-525.

Siefert, K., Bowman, P., Heflin, C., Danziger, S., and Williams, D. (2000). Social and environmental predictors of maternal depression in current and recent welfare recipients. *American Journal of Orthopsychiatry*, 70: 510-522.

Siefert, K., Heflin, C.M., Corcoran, M.D., and Williams, D. (2001). Food insufficiency and the physical and mental health of low-income women. *Women and Health*, 32: 159-177.

Warner, V., Weissman, M.M., Mufson, L., and Wickramaratne, P.J. (1999). Grandparents, parents, and grandchildren at high risk for depression: A three-generation study. *Journal of the American Academy of Child & Adolescent Psychiatry*, 38: 289-296.

Williams, D.R., Yu, Y., Jackson, J.S., and Anderson, N.B. (1997). Racial differences in physical and mental health: Socioeconomic status, stress, and discrimination. *Journal of Health Psychology*, 2: 335-351.

## Author's Notes

The author wishes to thank Professors Kristine Siefert, Sheldon Danziger, Carol Mowbray, and Assistant Dean for Research, Kenneth Lutterman at the University of Michigan School of Social Work for their comments and suggestions. The author also wishes to thank Nili Tannenbaum for her substantive editorial contributions to this paper.

# Health and Mental Health Disparities Among Black Americans

**James S. Jackson, Ph.D.***
**Institute for Social Research**
**University of Michigan**

## Introduction

Disparities in living conditions and socio-economic resources, and variations in socio-cultural factors between African Americans and non-blacks, contribute to ethnic and racial differences in health and mental health statuses and services. The accumulated research data argue for the importance of race, ethnicity, and socio-cultural factors in forming both the context and sources of important influences on normal development as well as for the nature, expression, and course of mental disorder (Jackson, 1990).

Unfortunately, these contextual factors have been viewed largely as nuisance variation in much research. Given their importance in understanding basic cognitive, social, and pathological processes, greater attention must be placed on studying these factors in the course of both "normal" human development and psychopathology for minority groups. This research agenda provides the scholarly and conceptual foundations for the work underway in the African American Mental Health Research Program (AAMHRP).

Our prior research suggests that disparities between African and non-African Americans in resources and environmental stressors contribute to critical differences in access to treatment, diagnosis, assignment to certain types of treatments, dropping out of treatment (premature termination) and treatment outcome (Neighbors, Jackson, Campbell and Williams, 1989). More research is needed in the areas of epidemiology (true prevalence), documentation of unmet service needs, as well as studies of the impact of culturally specific treatment interventions on increasing use, decreasing treatment dropout and increasing the probability of successful outcome. In conducting effective cross-cultural clinical interventions, there is preliminary evidence that cultural knowledge of African Americans is a necessary, but insufficient, "first step". Knowledge of culture alone cannot replace the necessity of providing adequate service delivery systems, high quality therapeutic skills and effective follow-up.

## Ethnic Disparities in Use of Mental Health Services

Although the reported rates for diagnosed mental illness for African

American and non-blacks are comparable, the access and utilization of mental health services are very different. The disparities are most notable in the under-utilization of outpatient services by African Americans and the over-representation of African Americans in inpatient facilities.

Under or non-utilization of services is a problem for ethnic minorities, especially when service access is viewed in relation to the prevalence of psychiatric morbidity in the general population (U.S. Department of Health and Human Services, 2001). Given the fact that ethnic minorities are an increasing proportion of the nation's population, this issue will be increasingly significant. Some explanations for minority under-utilization are well documented; one explanation for black under-utilization is the stigma attached to seeking mental health help. Another is that African Americans are more likely to use alternative informal support systems or indigenous practitioners (Neighbors & Jackson, 1984). A third explanation for black under-utilization is that African Americans hold negative attitudes toward psychotherapy and mental health services. It has also been argued that therapists are uncomfortable in treating the low-income, black client and as a result, blacks are less likely to be accepted for treatment (Lewis, 1991). Finally, because black Americans are disproportionately represented among the poor, they are more likely to obtain mental health help from the public mental health care sector. As a result, minorities are seen less often, over a shorter period of time, and are more likely to receive drug therapy in comparison to those receiving private mental health (Knesper, 1985). This finding also means that blacks are more likely to be found in treatment modalities characterized by low intervention (i.e., categorical treatment such as alcohol, substance abuse, or chronic units) and paraprofessional staff (Mollica, Blum & Redlich, 1980).

However, the literature on the under-utilization of mental health services by ethnic minorities suffers from the lack of an epidemiologic database required to document the true need for mental health services among African Americans.

Historically, the research findings have confirmed that minority status is highly correlated with likelihood of dropout from mental health facilities. In fact, premature termination of treatment has long been the cornerstone of the argument that traditional mental health services are inadequate for minorities. More recent studies by Mollica *et al.* (1980), O'Sullivan *et al.* (1989) and Snowden *et al.* (1989) all indicate that in the 10-20 years since the launching of the Community Mental Health Movement access for under-represented minorities has increased. In one case (Mollica, 1980), it seemed clear that a new community mental health center had improved service delivery to ethnic groups previously denied entry in to anything but the state hospital. This heightened utilization pattern is consistent with national data reported by Chung (1986) on the use of community mental health centers by minorities since the Community Mental Health Centers Act. A decrease in the minority dropout rates was reported by O'Sullivan (1989) and Snowden (1989). They suggest that an increase in cultural compatibility could account for these improvements. However, further studies are needed to more clearly document this hypothesis (Snowden & Cheung), 1990.

Racial matching of patient and therapist is a complicated and highly charged issue. Some studies find a clear preference for an ethnically matched therapist. Other studies found no ethnic differences in preference for type of therapy, patient satisfaction or degree of self disclosure, that depended on the ethnicity of the therapist. Jones and Matsumoto (1982) argue that the time has come to move beyond focusing exclusively on race and social class to investigation of the actual mediating factors that prevent successful therapeutic work. In their view social class and ethnicity are only proxies for other variables affecting the interpersonal relationship and, as proxies, they fail to inform us about what truly makes therapy successful. For example, meaningful knowledge of culture emerges as an important but not exclusive tool whereby the culturally different therapist can achieve credibility and effective therapy.

Very little current research has focused on the evaluation of treatment outcomes in minority populations. Based on current data, therapist characteristics like warmth, empathy, and honesty would seem to be highly important determinants of patient improvement regardless of racial, ethnic, or cultural identity. There is little empirical research that addresses, directly, the treatment effectiveness of specific modalities or the relative efficacy of different treatment approaches to different ethnic groups.

Sue (1988) cites the following methodological limitations on outcome research with minorities: the race of clients and therapists have not been fully matched; there is a lack of random assignment to treatment and control groups; the small numbers of subjects used in most studies result in low statistical power; socioeconomic status is confounded with race because this variable is often not controlled; and, many studies are correlational in nature and thus cannot provide information about causal issues. Thus, the only real consensus is that not enough outcome research on minorities has been conducted and much of what has been done suffers from methodological problems.

At our institute, we are studying discrete mental disorders and their pathways into treatment, diagnostic divergence, and treatment efficacy and treatment outcomes. We believe that there is clearly a need for research that assesses risk factors, individual and family strengths, individual psychopathology and service use all within a context that addresses a focus on multiple (individual, family, community, organizational) levels of research and analysis.

The finding is that blacks may be more likely to use mental health services currently than they were in the 1950's and 1960's; yet it seems clear that they are still not using mental health services as much as their clinically-defined needs, based on what more sophisticated epidemiologic studies would indicate. One can only conclude that there remain substantial barriers to mental health services utilization that must be overcome (U.S. Department of Health and Human Services, 2001).

## Mental Health Status

In the 1980's, the National Institute of Mental Health, by supporting the National Survey of Black Americans (NSBA) (Jackson, 1991), recognized the importance of obtaining nationally representative data on the mental and physical health of one of America's major minority groups, African Americans. Today, the NIMH is supporting three very large national populations surveys, the National Survey of American Life (NSAL) and the National Latino and Asian American Surveys (NLAAS), that will provide unprecedented current national data on the major minority populations, and a significant number of subgroups within these populations. The proposed study will contain a sample size that is five times larger with adequate representation of non-Hispanic Caribbean blacks as well as important demographic sub-groups within both the African American and Caribbean black samples. Similar large numbers and differentiated sub-groups will also be available on Latino and Asian groups in NLAAS.

With the exceptions of schizophrenia and phobias the ECA found roughly comparable rates of mental disorders for blacks and whites

(Robins & Regier, 1991). For example, age-adjusted analyses by sex and ECA site did not show any consistent black excess in lifetime or six-month prevalence of depression (Somervell *et al.*, 1989). Even more striking, results from the National Comorbidity Study (NCS) found that rates of disorders for African Americans were consistently below those of whites; these differences were particularly pronounced for depression and substance abuse disorders (Blazer *et al.*, 1994; Kessler *et al.*, 1994). The only exception to this trend was in the rates of phobia, where blacks had slightly, but significantly, higher rates of agoraphobia than whites (Magee *et al*, 1996). Closer inspection of the NCS data revealed further complexity; black women had higher current rates of agoraphobia and simple phobia than white women. Black men, however, had rates of simple and social phobia that were two and three times lower than white men (Magee, 1993).

The NCS prevalence estimates of mental disorder were substantially above those reported in the ECA (Kessler *et al.*, 1996). These findings raise important issues about the reliability of diagnoses using structured survey instruments and their ability to predict the need for clinical treatment. Meeting standard clinical criteria alone may no longer be sufficient for identifying cases in community studies; it has been suggested that the level of impairment must also be considered (Regier *et al.*, 1996). Approaches to the measurement of the degree of impairment associated with mental disorder have a long tradition in psychiatric epidemiology (Langner & Michael, 1963; Strole *et al.*, 1962). Combining impairment with diagnostic criteria makes it possible to reassess the concept of "caseness" (Neighbors, 1984; Richman & Barry, 1985; Sachs-Ericsson & Ciarlo, 1992). In the new studies extensive assessment of impairment, independent of specific disorders and severity will be available.

## Conceptual Orientation: Stress and Adaptation Model

Historically, the work at Michigan has employed a stress, coping, and social resource model to guide data collection, analyses and interpretation (Jackson *et al.*, 1986). In the NSBA, and twenty years later in the ongoing National Survey of American Life (NSAL), we are using a stress and adaptation approach to understanding the distribution of distress and disorders among African Americans and other minority groups (Pearlin, 1989; Pearlin *et al.*, 1981). The life-stress paradigm provides a useful framework for considering and understanding the role of stressors in the lives of blacks and other discriminated— against groups. Outlined in terms of this framework, the ongoing research 1) examines the nature and distribution of stressors and stress among major minority groups and whites by important structural and sociodemographic factors; 2) examines the influence of these stressors on mental disorders, severity, psychological distress, and impairment; and 3) explores the role of psychological and social resources (*e.g.*, mastery, self-esteem, informal emotional and instrumental support, religious involvement, etc.) in buffering the effects of stress on mental health and help-seeking.

Specifically, this work focuses on the relative importance of race, ethnicity, socioeconomic status (SES) and gender, as well as factors like acculturation, as antecedents for understanding the nature of stress and its influences, for example, on mental health and services used by those with mental disorders. Just as an example of the needed subtlety of defining and assessing potential mediating and moderation factors, we recognize that the effects of SES must be assessed not only at the level of the individual and household but also at the level of the neighborhood (*e.g.*, Krieger *et al.*, 1997). Regardless of individual or household characteristics, black, white, Latino, Caribbean and Asian neighborhoods differ dramatically in their availability of jobs, crime levels, family structures, opportunities for marriage, and exposure to conventional role models (*e.g.* Wilson 1987; 1996).

One critical issue is the extent to which minority status increases risk for health and mental health problems (*e.g.* Vega & Rumbaut, 1991; Williams & Fenton, 1994; Aneshenel, 1992). For example, previous research has long argued that discrimination per se adversely affects the mental health of African Americans (*e.g.* McCarthy & Yancey, 1971). However, stressors that may be unique to, or more prevalent among, African Americans have been incorporated into the assessment of stress (Jackson, *et al.*, 1996; McLean & Link, 1994; Pearlin, 1989; Essed, 1991; Feagin, 1991). Several studies indicate that racial discrimination, as measured by subjective reports, adversely affects the emotional well-being (and physical health outcomes such as blood pressure) of African Americans and other minorities (*e.g.* Salgado de Snyder, 1987(; Armaro *et al.*, 1987; Saldana, 1995; Jackson *et al.*, 1996; Williams & Chung, 1997; James *et al.*, 1984; Krieger, 1990; Krieger & Signey, 1996). Other evidence suggests that the experience of unfair treatment, irrespective of race or ethnicity, may have negative consequences for health (Harburg *et al.*, 1973).

Our ongoing research will identify the types and amounts of discrimination that affect mental health and will allow us to begin to explain how racial/ethnic bias combines with other types of stress to affect mental health among the heterogeneous minority populations. Particular attention will be given to the recency, timing, frequency, and cumulative impact of experiencing incidents of bias.

Exposure to stress does not always adversely affect mental health (Cohen *et al.*, 1995). Social support and psychological resources that can mitigate the impact of stress on health include positive social relationships, self-esteem, perceptions of mastery or control, self-regulation of anger or hostility, and capacity for repression or denial of unwelcome emotions such as feelings of helplessness or hopelessness (House *et al.*, 1988; Kessler *et al.*, 1995; Mirowsky & Ross, 1989; Rogler *et al.*, 1989; Mirowsky & Ross, 1980; Williams, 1990; Williams & Fenton, 1994). Analyses of data from a 1995 Detroit Area Study highlight the importance of understanding the nature of the coping processes (Williams *et al.*, 1997). In that study, the mental health outcomes of blacks exceeded that of whites, when adjusted for the effects of race-related stress. This pattern is consistent with the suggestion that stressful experiences may more adversely affect the mental health of whites than blacks. Kessler (1979) documented a similar pattern for the relationship between stressful life events and psychological distress for nonwhites (mainly blacks).

A broad range of other coping resources, including family support and religious involvement, play an important role in buffering minority populations from the negative effects of stress. Prior research suggests that religion can have a positive impact on psychological well-being by providing systems of meaning that help individuals make sense of stressful experiences. Further, involvement in religious communities can be an important source of social integration and social support (*e.g.* Taylor & Chatters, 1988; Williams, 1994). The data now being collected will permit, in a more thorough study than has previously been done, analyzing how religious beliefs, behavior, and experiences combine with other social and psychological resources to influence the individual responses to stressful experience.

Epidemiological research focusing on group differences across populations in psychopathology and within-group differences among racial/ethnic minorities is particularly important given the precarious economic and social situations of many minority Americans. Despite the impressive advances in knowledge concerning the national distributions of psychopathology, the prevalence of psychological distress, and help-seeking behavior and mental health service use, our knowledge of serious mental disorders and mental health among and within minority sub-group populations remain meager. Our current research will provide a broader assessment of risk factors and adaptive resources than previous work, including the assessment of unique stressors and resources that affect the minority populations.

## Implications for Training and Education

There is a clear and urgent need to translate the remarkable advances of neuroscience and the biomedical sciences into the education and training of the full spectrum of professionals engaged in the delivery of mental health services.

At the same time, there is a less well recognized but equally compelling need to also incorporate the research findings of the behavioral and social sciences concerning poverty, racism and cultural attributes, as major factors in contributing to the occurrence of mental disorder as well as the probability of successful treatment.

Given the large and growing population of minorities, this aspect of mental health will be increasingly important. There is evidence that minority groups do not receive adequate care despite the fact that their needs are great. There is a body of research that, if taught to the relevant mental health professionals, can help them to reduce an important source of the disparities in the delivery of mental health services for minorities. There is a need for heightened efforts to recruit minority practitioners in all of the mental health related professions. However, regardless of the ethnicity or race of the therapist, there is a body of knowledge that should be taught concerning the range of barriers to quality mental health services for minorities along with the fundamentals of an evidence-based understanding of the psychotherapeutic needs of ethnic and racially diverse patients.

Although much is now known, there is also a need for continuing research to fill the gaps in the understanding of treatment outcomes for minorities. As a result, there should also be an emphasis on research training for continuing studies in the area of mental health disparities in addition to the focus on the education and training practitioners.

There is a need for greater interdisciplinary training of psychiatrists and the other mental health professionals. Newer, more effective mental health services will require coordinated, comprehensive interdisciplinary delivery systems that will coordinate agencies and professional disciplines. Therefore, the comprehensive education and training of mental health service professionals will also require greater attention to the interdisciplinary training and supervised learning of how to work in these newer, more effective settings.

This new approach to education and training of mental health professionals can play a vital role in achieving greater equality and effectiveness in meeting the mental health needs of a diverse American society.

---

* *This paper represents a summary of a longer paper which was prepared for this conference by Dr. Jackson. The full paper and all references may be obtained at the following address:*

James S. Jackson
426 Thompson Street
P.O.B. 1248
University of Michigan
Ann Arbor, MI 48106-1248

e-mail: jamessj@umich.edu

## Challenges in Healthcare: Latinos

**David J. Sanchez, Jr., Ph.D.,**
**University of California — San Francisco**

The nation's fastest growing population, the Latino, encompasses many diverse subcultures: Puerto Rican, Cuban, Mexican, Dominican, Central American, and South American, among others. Key variables, such as proximity to Latin American language, core culture, religion and economics, with a continuum of migration back and forth from the host country, are as prevalent today as a century ago.

My grandparent and parents came from Mexico and Nicaragua in the mid-1910s to the port city of San Francisco, California. To migrant families, urban life offered jobs in trade, shipping, transportation, the textile industries, meat packing companies, (butcher towns), and steel and chemical plants, or as day laborers. The Latino community then was largely Mexican and Catholic. Some were recent migrants, who came for reasons such as political revolutions, or God, Gold and Glory. Yet some had been here in the 1800s when California was still under the rule of Spain and Mexico.

During this period, as my family began to adjust, the community experienced illness and disease. The flu epidemic exploded, but there was also tuberculosis, anxiety and depression, posttraumatic stress disorders, alcoholism and emerging mental health problems. Given the unique needs of this population, treatment was limited. Access, language, diagnosis and treatment, and comprehensive follow-up were not valid models at that point in time.

Today there are nearly 40 million Latinos within the United States. The majority resides in urban areas, though there are now significant numbers in rural communities. Everywhere there is considerable diversity. In the San Francisco area, for example, many Latinos are from Central America, Mexico, the Caribbean, and South America. The diversity of subcultures is significant as core groups bring unique languages to communities and often find limited access to basic health care and mental services.

Diversity poses a significant challenge to the health care system. At San Francisco General Hospital over 45 languages are spoken daily. In New York City, Chicago, Atlanta, Miami, Boston, more than 60 languages are spoken. Even in states such as North Carolina, Wisconsin, Iowa, Kentucky, and Georgia, the number of Latinos is growing. Some medical schools, such as Wake Forest, are beginning to address this challenge by implementing Spanish courses for medicine and nursing students.

As the migration continues, reinforced by geography, media, proximity, and languages, the desire for good jobs, housing, and schools, survival of the core family remains the hope and dream of many. Some of the health needs and challenges of the past persist, but now they are joined by other problems, by asthma, cancer, high blood pressure, diabetes, growing numbers of those with substance abuse and HIV, the community epidemic of gang violence and warfare, and the reoccurrence of infectious diseases such as tuberculosis.

The Latino community continues to focus on young people and to emphasize the importance of extended family and of dignity and respect for one's elders but acculturations tends to dilute these values and public education may even be viewed as a barrier by some members of the community. This seems to be a significant factor in the rise of mental health illness for the community. In the Los Angeles school district more than 45% of students are Latino; and schools in other areas, in Seattle and San Jose, for instance, and in parts of the Northeast, the South and the Midwest are showing great increases in numbers of Spanish speaking students. However, at 50%, the number of dropouts from this cohort is the highest in the nation.

In higher education, we see a limited number of Latino students admitted, and even fewer graduated and continuing on to professional schools such as medicine and nursing. At the faculty level, Latinos comprise less than 5% of the faculty in all health professional schools. These barriers have been here for too long and must be removed to ensure that our national health care system will provide adequate culturally/linguistically competent health providers for the rich diversity of this nation.

The public health system and its collaborations with non-profit agencies that serve so many of our refugee and immigrant populations has been key to providing care for these groups. In San Francisco, mental health services offered to diverse populations through the Department of Public Health reflect true partnerships and collaborations, which have evolved to assure the highest quality or care for our families.

And now, through the public schools, new wellness centers have developed pathways with our culturally focused mental health units. This integration of services through the community, school and hospitals is beginning to make a difference. The integrated service model is now available to our law enforcement agencies for pre-service and training of both senior and recruit personnel and the Department of Public Health is involved in training within our prison system. The dropout rate for Latinos cited earlier is almost directly linked to our overrepresentation in the penal system, both juvenile and adult.

The continuum of care and the continuum of migration bring to our health care systems great opportunities to design and develop multiple systems based on our unique areas of service. We need to increase access to our mental health system and be inclusive in its service areas. We need to expand community-based alternatives, forge new pathways and improve integration of services, especially for non-English speaking families that may require multiple services. We need to strengthen our multi-cultural basic prevention programs and activities and to sustain and expand community partnerships based on measured outcomes and quality control. Given limited resources, we must maximize opportunities to strengthen infrastructures and ensure the level of training and supervision for new personnel and exemplary continuing in-service education for our senior health professionals and non-certified staff.

I have full confidence we are all up for this challenge. Our numbers may not be overwhelming but our mission is steadfast: to ensure that diverse Latino populations will have access, along with all Americans, to an effective and culturally competent community-based mental health system. Our pathways may differ but our commitment to access and quality care with this multi-cultural model will make a difference.

## Discussion Highlights, Session IV

### Disparities

— A body of evidence suggests there is racial bias, whatever the source, in both the choice of diagnosis and, more strongly, in the choice of treatment for different conditions. There are also variations in seeking of care for depression and other symptoms of mental disorder. The most well studied area of racial differentials is cardiac treatment where, even when such other factors as insurance coverage and socio-economic status were considered, race was the only differential that mattered. Physicians need to understand that there are racial differences in the way care is provided.

— A retreat from the community by clinical medicine and even public health has abandoned the "people in the trenches," the social workers and school counselors who are not trained in an advanced way but are trying to hold things together. Leaders who understand how knowledge and socio-economic conditions can affect people's lives are needed. At this point no one goes into communities to do basic work, to gain knowledge of underlying pathophysiology and genetics and to understand how community forces affect both individual families and communities. Those people are needed to advocate for change in the way society is structured and to find ways to eliminate underlying disparities. There will always be need for good clinicians, but also for psychiatrists who understand how communities are organized and how they work, what a healthy community looks like and how to engage people.

— Physical and mental health are strongly correlated with race, ethnicity, and poverty. The question is why? Is it the environment or the quality of care which has been demonstrated to be poor? Black people get less anesthesia than white. Is the health care delivery system in the wrong place, since much psychiatric care is provided after the fact in jail? Is it the insensitivity of those who don't understand cultural backgrounds or different languages? Why do Latino patients go through interviews with people who don't understand the Spanish language?

— Hispanics will comprise about 26% of the population in the next few decades, becoming the largest minority. But this is not a monolithic group, for 64% are of Mexican origin, and they live mainly in the west; 18% are Puerto Ricans and they are found in the northeast; 8% are Cubans who live mostly in Florida. The remainder are South American and Caribbean, found in many parts of the country. The fact that Hispanic communities are now emerging in different parts of the country creates a challenge for demographers and for meeting public health needs.

— The heterogeneity of the Hispanic population requires research in both epidemiology and clinical areas, as well as in differences between old and new Hispanic communities. One study found that the prevalence of severe mental illness differs in Mexicans Compared to Mexican Americans, who have a higher rates of depression, psychosis and substance abuse, comparable to the rest of the population, immigrants born in Mexico have rates comparable to those found in Mexico City. Understanding how Americanization affects second and third generations is important for both research and the provision of services.

— The Hispanic workforce remains an important issue. The number of Hispanic medical students has increased very little in the past few dacades while the number of Hispanic psychiatric residents has remained flat, compared with the growth of Asian-Americans in those fields, which is impressive. The number of Hispanic psychiatric nurses and social workers is very low as is the number of Hispanic faculty members, which is about 5% overall but 11% in the southwest.

— More Hispanics need to be attracted to the health professions, but there is also a need to increase the cultural competence of other health care workers to improve familiarity with the culture and language and the use of interpreters to respond to the needs of this growing population.

— Issues related to culture and ethnicity are important to health outcomes. Clinicians who are well-intentioned and want to improve health need to be trained to be more sensitive to cultural differences, much as they are trained to be sensitive to different personal attributes. In the realm of public health, research is needed to provide adequate information on ethnic subgroups and their needs. The suggestion is being made that evidence-based methods tested mostly in white populations ought to be tried with members of ethnic subgroups, but it would be better first to have specific information about those subgroups.

— Some people say race is not important and that ethnicity is what matters: but where so much history is based on race, it is hard to ignore. What it means to be in a category called "black" in the United States is profoundly different than to be in a category called "white." The finding that race, not socio-economic status, is more important in the kind of health care that is provided has another dimension. Even when services are provided, the probability is high that people providing the services are not as good, that even when a by-pass operation is provided to an African-American, the surgeon is likely to have higher mortality rates.

— Emergency room studies suggest that stereotypes tend to emerge under stress. Stereotypes do come from a larger social and cultural context but they impact individual exchanges. As the nation becomes more diverse, stereotypes will be more of a problem for individual interactions than they are now.

— While tremendous disparities are seen in health, large disparities are not seen with regard to mental disorders. There are, however, huge disparities in treatment. One possible explanation for the small disparities with mental disorders but the great health disparities may be that the idea of losing one's mind is so horrible that people do almost anything to escape, even engaging in behaviors damaging to health. One way to preserve one's life may be to drink a lot, but that's not going to help with health outcomes.

— Stereotyping of groups must be avoided but at the same time demographic issues and distinct population differences must be considered in the delivery of care. It is also important to be aware of the need to change the demography of the health care professions workforce. Changing that demography will require close collaboration with education to develop the pipeline of students into professional schools. By the time students reach medical school it is too late to change the demographic composition.

— The only developed country where there is evidence that children's problems are getting worse is the United States. Increasing disparities in income and socio-economic status accounts for much of the increase in children's problems.

— Though the conference was designed to say that a substantial body of knowledge is being inadequately applied on a day-to-day basis, it instead disclosed a welter of exhaustive and challenging problems. It is important to focus on what role a foundation can play and not try to do too much. Exciting as genome or new findings in molecular biology may be, they offer no current likelihood of benefit. While information of psychotherapies may warrant wider use, they are not a cure-all. It is also important to respect those on the front line and allow them to do the best they can with the knowledge they have.

— It is possible that strengthing individual functions, talents and capacities may have a modifying effect on either the frequency or nature of dysfunction. Education seems to be a protective factor against the development of Alzheimer's disease. Children respond eagerly to the program of books in pediatricians' offices. Concern about drop-outs led to a program to help attach them to institutions and give them goals. In an effort to moderate the extraordinary amount of social dysfunction, and the soft and hard illnesses in the society, perhaps models drawing on such findings should be developed to enhance, encourage and facilitate the functioning of an individual to provide a broader sense of value to society.

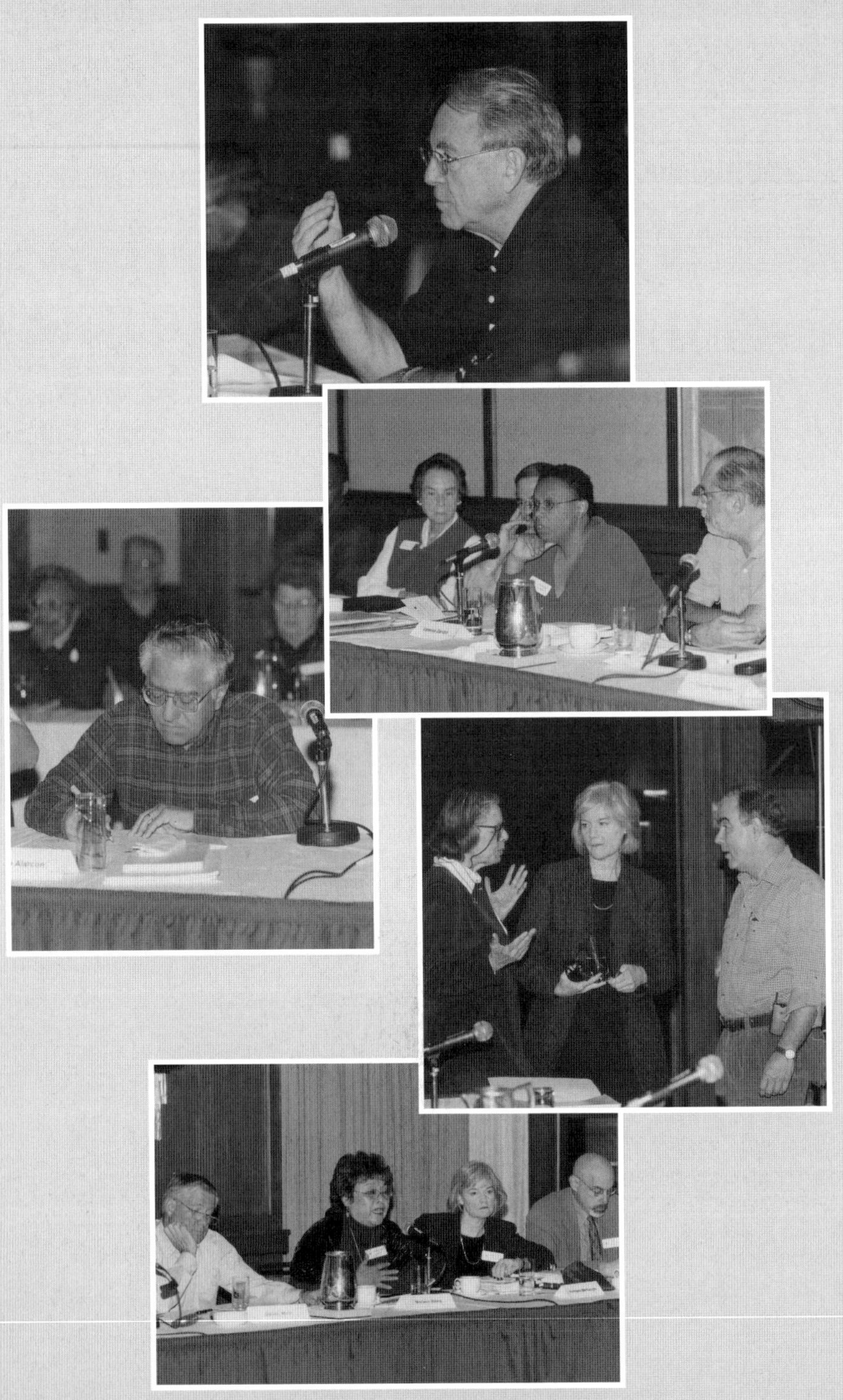

# Session V

## Conclusions and Recommendations

*Dr. Herbert Pardes opened the session with an invited summary and overview of the conference. The text of these remarks is printed here. The rest of the final session was devoted to participant comments, conclusions and recommendations based on their reflections on the proceedings of the entire conference. This process generated the following recommendations.*

## Conference Overview

**Herbert Pardes, M.D.,**
**Columbia Presbyterian Medical Center**

### There are many salient questions.

*What's the problem? The problem starts with the fact that mental health and substance abuse needs are not being met. The next question that could be raised is why is that true? Are the needs so overwhelming, given the fact that the needs are so intimately tied to other social problems? Are they overwhelming because there have been such cuts in resources and reimbursement?*

*Why do people not use the research that's there? Are they biased? Not listening? Not reading to keep up with what's going on? Is the research not helpful enough? Are people poorly trained? Is training bad? Are teachers closed-minded, outdated, turf-minded? How do we educate and prepare future mental health professionals?*

*Do we have adequate numbers of providers with the right skills? Do we have adequate numbers of the right resources? Do we suffer from the fact that people are simply using poor therapeutics or is it really all of the above and perhaps more? Do issues differ depending on which set of mental health and substance abuse problems you are talking about? Are you talking about the elderly or about children? Are you talking about co-morbidity, about alcohol or drugs? Nothing is homogeneous. The providers are not homogeneous, the illnesses are not homogeneous, and the age groups are not homogeneous. We have a number of cultures.*

*I can't cover the depth and breadth of this conference. We read excellent papers and heard a lot of excellent presentations. But I want to comment about this field. We have to remember where we came from, remember people being burned, and put in asylums and shackles. That was mental health for a number of centuries. Little by little people became more humanistic and attention was paid to people who were suffering as individuals. The psychoanalytic movement brought attention to listening to people, to trying to create some kind of individual, caring paradigm for the delivery of services.*

*Certainly the psychoanalytic movement was vulnerable due to the fact that sufficient science was not built up and many of the research enterprises were frustrated because it was difficult to prove or refute any kind of proposition. Many would criticize the fact that therapists would increasingly try to take care of people who didn't necessarily have the most severe illnesses while a large number of psychotic patients flowed through from city hospital to state hospitals and back out again, occasionally given shock therapy or some sedative. I do not have to read to know this history. I was there so I know what it was like.*

*As we trace rapidly through the 50s, 60s and 70s, in came things like deinstitutionalization. One thing that is very important is to pay attention to the field of psychopharmacology, which steadily over the years built a knowledge base and a set of treatments, which have had tremendous effect on the mental health field.*

*Also pertinent was the era of the community mental health movement, which had a wonderful philosophy and lasted for about 20 years. It was set aside in the late 70s and then, in a definitive way by the Reagan block grant programs in 1981.*

*The awareness of medications that might be helpful, a move to make mental health delivery more therapeutic, led also to the development of general hospital psychiatry as state hospital sectors began  to shut down. This was accompanied by a tremendous shift from inpatient to outpatient care. Mental health was one of the first medical areas to make that shift. Like it or not the mental health field was one of the first ones to introduce the idea of multidisciplinary involvement in clinical service. That stimulated a build up of mental health training programs in nursing, in s ocial work, in psychology as well as in some of the mental health primary care programs. This is not a new issue.*

*In the 80s, the big excitement was around brain science. That increased over the next twenty years. Think of findings that got attention. Recognition that the two brain hemispheres were different. Work that demonstrated deoxyglucose could be used to measure brain function through PET scans. Work by Eric Kandel on learning and memory for which he received the Lasker and then the Nobel Prize. Also included was work on neurotransmitters and on the MRI. All of this is exciting but these are not the only sciences of great consequence. There's also excitement about epidemiology because you need classification, you need diagnosis. This field started to develop some structure.*

*And then government. I was director of National Institute of Mental Health (NIMH) three years in the Carter Administration and three in Reagan. I only can say they were different. Federal grant programs for community mental health and substance became block programs, and if Congress during the Reagan Administration hadn't put strings on it, we wouldn't have anything.*

*A number of good things happened. Stigma declined. The citizen advocacy movement grew in the 80s. That was a wonderful development, one of the most important developments in the history of the field. Advocacy for parity started. It recently has become more of a drumbeat. Celebrities came out in greater numbers, acknowledging they were patients and had psychiatric illness. All this, and the fact that there were better therapeutics and better regard for research came together to give a more positive view of mental health. Mental health is far better than it was years ago, but nobody would doubt that it has a long way to go.*

*What can one say about the field vintage 2001? Certainly that there are more treatments and they are better. That's one of the reasons for a more positive view. One of the nice things about mental health research is that it is not as sequestered as it used to be. In the 60s, psychiatry was always "over there". Today psychiatry and mental health are mainstream in terms of research, and also because of recognition of the extraordinary prevalence of mental health disorders.*

*It has been pointed out that by 2020, psychiatry would be 15 percent of the total burden of all illnesses. That means there is a lot of psychiatric need out there. It is worldwide. If you asked most people about most important health needs in the world, they would say nutrition and infectious diseases. I'm not sure they would come to the conclusion that psychiatric and mental health needs are as widespread as the data demonstrated. Then you have the Surgeon General telling us only 10-20% of those who need it are receiving care. That's not entirely new either. I remember hearing that 20 years ago.*

*There is hard research emphasizing diagnosis and treatment and also producing evidence for psychosocial treatment. Then there's genetics, immunology, imaging, but when you get down to it, the amount of immediate application to mental health and substance abuse problems from the research is still somewhat limited. There are no lab tests.*

*Yet there is justification for being optimistic. Steve Hyman commented about this notion of a modifiable brain. There was a time when the dogma was you had a brain, that was it. That's history. We know the brain is responsive to environmental changes and new neurons actually have been produced. That's very encouraging, but it doesn't enable me to take care of a patient this afternoon.*

*And we need more research on dual diagnosis. We need a child psychiatric research agenda. How do you do this in a way that takes advantage of the multiple disciplines in research? Research needs multiple disciplines. One caution with all this excitement about research is that, in the excitement about the brain, genes, and the mechanics, we not forget the humanistic and psychosocial.*

*In 1981, the federal government decided to leave the services arena. We went to the Office of Management and Budget (OMB) in '81 or '82 and figured one thing we could do would be at least to evaluate the results of pulling out of mental health services. We were told that's not our concern.*

*Subsequent to that, we had the introduction of managed care, with the decimation of a good part of the health system. Anybody looking at the data knows mental health was particularly badly slashed by managed care. Now we have a push for parity on one side while reimbursement is being cut on the other side. We have the safety net disrupted, and the education system in bad shape. How do you specify need? Prevalence estimates don't necessarily equate to need. How do you define the right level of use? In substance abuse, you find a lot of co-morbidity and also a high incidence of recurrence.*

*We have better ways of dealing with this but the encouragement of for-profit centers has led to decimation of psychiatric services. Despite the fact that we have exciting research, we don't have all the answers. And at the end of the day, those who do clinical work have to go back and take care of patients.*

*Regarding psychosocial therapy, it is encouraging that there is more evidence on the table. That's been sorely needed. With a 20- to 30-year history of arguments with the Senate Finance Committee, one of the things needed was evidence. It is starting to come, but for the bulk of psychotherapy that is delivered there's still not the kind of evidence that's needed. Getting people outside the field to do evaluation studies so that we know what we are dealing with is important.*

*But beyond that, we have a school system which is a* de facto *mental health system for children. We have all kinds of other systems involved in the delivery of mental health, e.g. the justice system. Psychiatrists cannot do it all. Certainly that is not new, so we have got to pay attention to other professionals. When you do, you have to satisfy yourself that the nature of training they are getting and their abilities to deal with the range of problems matches the challenges they are going to experience.*

*Studies of the treatment and diagnostic patterns of general practitioners have not been very encouraging, particularly with psychotherapy. The wrong diagnosis, wrong medications, every conceivable error that could be made was made, and made in great numbers. This notion of "let's just train the general docs and they'll take care of it" is not easy. I can say that for a lot of these issues. Each of these issues could have a special conference.*

*But there is no question that we need multiple professionals to deliver mental health care. We have to figure out how to prepare them and ensure how what the patient ultimately receives is worth receiving. Currently the mental health-primary care relationship is in tatters.*

*The value of evidence-based therapies, in greater numbers and with more information, is clear. And we have got to give credit to psychopharmacologists. Over the years, they've laid out a steady record of progress. The result is a range of therapies which have dramatically changed the field. Observations about the value of lithium have provided one of the most important therapeutic developments in the mental health field.*

*The attention to encouraging more integration between population-based approaches and individual clinical approaches, and the integration between pharmacological or biological approaches and the psychosocial, is important and yet very difficult. How do you develop teachers who genuinely integrate in caring for psychiatric patients a pharmacological and a psychosocial approach? We started to have two people train the residents, a psychosocial expert and a pharmacologist but who weaves it together? What it takes to do that is worth a conference.*

*Then there is a challenge to kinds of therapies that are sequestered. Do you bring in family? Do it in the school or in the house? Do you bring together education and mental health? It is an enormous job to separate different kinds of problems and determine the right approach for that problem. I'm not ready to sign off on the idea that every treatment should be done in this way. I think it is well taken that there are problems with existing therapies in regard to the way the child is treated and the family is shut out.*

*What are the training challenges? Where do you focus? On the numbers? We need multiple disciplines. There are too few child psychiatrists and, maybe, too few psychiatrists. Are there enough people going into the field that focus on biology and the brain?*

*On the nature of training, we're encouraged to provide more on evidence-based therapies to psychiatrists and, perhaps, others as well. We're also encouraged to give more training on the pharmacological products for non-medical professionals. We want to ensure adequacy of training for all disciplines. We also want to look at how to strengthen training for family care and primary care doctors as well as for mental health professionals beyond their training who may need education in evidence-based therapies. We applaud what we heard about credentials for geriatric psychiatry, but the need for geriatric care is vast. Who is going to deal with it?*

*How do you train consumers? To what extent would people knowing more about mental health themselves make them better consumers of mental health care? With children, it was commented that a study of a number of different countries showed the US was one in which problems for children have worsened in recent years. Do they take the brunt of changes in social philosophy? Are we reeling from the tendency in this country to walk away from people who have needs? As long as we have resources, do we let the other half make it as well as they can?*

*There is a shortage of child psychiatrists but who is it who are experts in adolescent psychiatry? Where do you go? One of the problems in child mental health involves classification and measurement of childhood disorders. The focus on the education system being in difficult shape goes along with the decline in social servic-*

*es, but we must not forget the impact of the media on children and the kinds of violence to which they are exposed.*

*Dual diagnosis is increasing in frequency, with the need for a range of services and more partial hospitalization. We need to emphasize the value of case management and the need for community housing and support. A set of additional needs has to be attended to if we want to give someone a chance. We need to look at illness, and then think in terms of housing, employment, finances, medical care, etc.*

*Cultural issues pervade every aspect. An approach to mental health and substance abuse can't be made without recognition of the cultural context. There are problems in diagnosis, therapy, and allocation of resources and services. This is a big issue in training. We want people out there who understand the context of the individual with whom they are working.*

*We also want adequate numbers so the provider group mirrors the recipient source. We need more students who represent the rich fabric of this country. Then we have the problem of trying to disentangle how much is cultural, how much is economic. And minority groups are not necessarily homogeneous. There are multiple subgroups of minority groups.*

*We should recommend a systematic look at therapies for different conditions. We could take populations and look at how services could be best organized. We could decide to get to leaders of training and talk about whether we can make training more responsive. We should try to lay out a concept as to how to decide the adequate kind of delivery given the prevalence. Should 100 percent of those diagnosed be receiving services? Do we need guidelines for functional disability to dictate which people who should be treated? Will we find that, if we don't have a defined concept, the demand and need will be so overwhelming that we can't get anywhere? We should focus on ways of increasing integration.*

*But let's be realistic about what a single foundation can do in this extraordinary complex of problems. Many wonderful reports grace shelves throughout the country. Do we focus on the policy agenda to strengthen the community mental health program? Or on a public health approach to problems of children's mental health? Should we pursue an agenda to increase the number of trainees? For years we fought the endless pressure to eliminate training and education in mental health.*

*Maybe we should be focusing on a policy that allows those who provide services to have more intensive or comprehensive training. Should we look at enhancing normal functions as a way of mitigating dysfunction? When we talked about Alzheimer's disease, it was pointed out that education is negatively correlated. Studies of the brain tell us that there's something positive about books and kids. Exercise helps to diminish arthritis. Should we try to attach youth to components of society, to give them a sense of involvement and worth? Some studies show a child involved in school is less likely to be involved in substance abuse.*

*One idea I like is reintegrating National Institute of Mental Health (NIMH), National Institute on Drug Abuse (NIDA) and National Institute on Alcohol Abuse and Alcoholism (NIAAA) with the respective service areas of the Substance Abuse and Mental Health Services Agency (SAMSA). Years ago the Senate had a hearing at which the Alcohol Drug Abuse and Mental Health Administration (ADAMHA) and National Institutes of Health (NIH) people tried to show that keeping research and services together had a value. Why didn't NIH do it? Some people who thought they had to sanitize mental health said the best way to do it would be to take the institutes and give them to NIH to give credibility. NIH is not focused on services. With the talk about translation of research to services, does it make sense to separate these entities?*

*We have got to decide what problem we want to attack, and lay out the scope of the problem. What can the Foundation do that will be useful? Does that involve this conference, or a set of additional conferences as well?*

*In summary, we don't want to minimize the extraordinary challenge in front of us but there's a tremendous amount that's been done in this field which represents real progress, whether it is the excitement of research or the fact that we have better therapeutics or the fact that we have more information coming along. There's a large body of people who are interested. The citizen group involvement is sensational.*

*We have an opportunity but also a big challenge. We have a political and philosophic fabric that's shifted markedly. That's going to be an uphill battle. Particularly how do we repair the system in light of September 11, which made people more aware that mental health services are valuable and drew the nation's attention to many of the bioterrorist issues? Now we have a nation in a chronic state of tension and mixtures of depression. Having said that, I would encourage us to try to make our report specific, to pick out the most important priorities and suggest whether that leads to additional activities.*

# Conclusions and Recommendations

**Conclusions:**

The timeliness and critical importance of the goal of enhancing the quality, supply and the diversity of the professional mental health workforce to meet new needs and to function in some new roles was affirmed unanimously. "We have the opportunity and the responsibility to redesign the way we train our future health professionals," one participant commented. Participants emphasized a number of essential core elements, among them mastering new evidence-based therapies; developing the attitudes and learning the skills for teamwork and collaboration across systems; recruitment of minority trainees; teaching respect for and knowledge of diverse cultural values; encouraging rigorous service research; and educating the public, consumer advocacy groups and policy makers about the availability and quality of mental health services.

Therefore, participants concluded that responsibility for implementing their recommendations rests with a wide spectrum of groups, agencies and individuals, including—but not limited to—academic health centers and training programs, professional organizations and societies, consumer advocacy and community groups, credentialing and licensing bodies, and the many local, state, and federal agencies concerned with the mental health of both individuals and communities.

They also recognized that carrying out this responsibility demands new working interfaces and collaboration among systems that currently operate alone. To create this new environment, they urged all parties to work together to identify and eliminate the full range of economic, institutional and "guild" barriers to achieving the goals implicit in the following recommendations.

**Recommendations:**

1. *Interdisciplinary Training and Collaboration:*

   **It is now clear that mental health services are best and most efficiently provided by an interdisciplinary team with a common, broad knowledge base. Therefore, all training should:**

   - include specific training curricula on the theory and skills of interdisciplinary collaboration;
   - create models of interdisciplinary treatment in clinical or practicum exercises;
   - develop joint programs across disciplines to provide interdisciplinary training to collaborating students;

- identify and reward faculty role models who participate in interdisciplinary professional education and patient care;
- utilize clinical settings that offer strong opportunities for teaching interdisciplinary care;
- and in all cases stress that the success of the collaboration will depend on mutual trust, respect and appreciation of each other's knowledge and skills to best benefit the patient.

2. *Evidence-based treatments* should be taught in all professional schools.

   For quality assurance, the mastery should be judged by performance criteria, not just the hours spent in taking the courses.

3. *Recruitment*— Given the existing shortage of professionals, an aggressive recruitment program must be developed to attract and train professionals in all the mental health disciplines.

   Particular emphasis must be placed on broadening representation from diverse racial, ethnic and cultural groups to serve their unmet needs. In addition, because the need is particularly acute, special effort must be given to recruiting and training more child and adolescent psychiatrists and other child mental health professionals.

4. *A common core curriculum* of mental health knowledge, skills and attitudes must be developed.

   This core curriculum should be taught across all medical specialties and to other mental health professionals to provide both a common vocabulary and an updated knowledge base among those who care for individuals and families. In addition to the formal teaching this core curriculum could be offered, updated and maintained as an Internet-based teaching module.

5. Community mental health must be revitalized by removing institutional barriers and developing stronger links across different systems, such as the public welfare, education and justice systems.

   Workers in those systems should be able to recognize mental illness and be able to identify the appropriate channels to provide care. A core curriculum of key concepts and skills in collaboration should be taught to this workforce.

6. *Public education* about the signs and symptoms and availability of effective treatment for mental disorders, as well as about the social costs incurred by not treating these disorders, is an important means of removing a significant barrier to the appropriate use of mental health services.

   For the general public, key concepts, as appropriate to all ages, cultural, ethnic/racial, and regional settings, should be provided on the Internet, possibly endorsed and maintained by NIMH, so that all Americans have access to reliable information about the diagnosis and treatment of common mental illnesses. Consumer advocacy groups and the media can be enlisted in public information programs.

7. *The prevention and treatment of mental health conditions* must include not only the individual but also the family and the community.

   Prevention and treatment must be tailored to specific demographic, socio-cultural, age, gender and ethnic contexts. Families and therapists must all be aware of the significance of these factors as related to a mental disorder.

8. *Credentialing and licensure.* Accreditation requirements and testing should include competence in the areas of collaboration, respect and understanding of diverse cultures, and mastery of all evidence-based therapies, including emphasis on the psychodynamic and cognitive.

   Whenever possible, officials will judge results using performance-based criteria rather than relying on the number of days or hours spent in didactic sessions. For example, documented reports of actual trainee time spent in inter-disciplinary contexts should be included.

Editor: Mary Hager
Design & production: Klaboe Design, New York
Cover design/photomontage: David Klaboe
Cover photos: Digital Vision & PhotoDisc: gettyimages.com
Conference photos: Matthew Glac, Fotografix, Toronto
Printed in USA by Cinnamon Graphics, Inc., New York